THE ENGLISH

YMCA
GUIDE TO
EXERCISE TO MUSIC

THE ENGLISH
YMCA
GUIDE TO
EXERCISE TO MUSIC

Rodney Cullum and Lesley Mowbray

PELHAM BOOKS
Stephen Greene Press

PELHAM BOOKS/Stephen Greene Press

Published by the Penguin Group
27 Wrights Lane, London W8 5TZ, England
Penguin USA, 375 Hudson Street, New York, NY 10014, USA
The Stephen Greene Press Inc., 15 Muzzey Street, Lexington, Massachusetts 02173, USA

Penguin Books Australia Ltd, Ringwood, Victoria, Australia
Penguin Books Canada Ltd, 2801 John Street, Markham, Ontario, Canada L3R 1B4
Penguin Books (NZ) Ltd, 182-190 Wairau Road, Auckland 10, New Zealand

Registered Offices: Harmondsworth, Middlesex, England

First published by Pelham Books 1986
Revised paperback edition 1988. Reprinted 1989, 1990

Copyright © Rodney Cullum and Lesley Mowbray 1986 and 1988

Filmset by Fakeham Photosetting Ltd, Norfolk
Printed and bound in Great Britain by Butler & Tanner Ltd, Frome and London

A CIP catalogue record for this book is available from the British Library

ISBN 0 7207 1851 I

DEDICATED TO   W. E. Lindley
                Bob and Iris
                Madge and Will

We would like to acknowledge the help, advice and support of:
Jill Benfield, Jenny Brown, Joanna Bryan, Alison Copeland,
Vernon Crew, Barry Cronin, Gary Doherty, Rex Hazeldene,
Colin Mawby, Huw Owen, Stephen Pain, Wayne Phillips, Steve
Saunders, Phillippa Ward and Steve Wooton.

Illustrations are by Alex Williams.

Contents

Foreword

Exercise to music has caught the imagination of many people now as a means of taking regular exercise. Its growth is of particular significance because many of the participants had not previously been attracted to any other forms of activity. However, the rapid increase in interest has created problems in that many of the current teachers have inadequate knowledge and expertise because of a lack of relevant training. Consequently their pupils are at risk when exercising under their instruction.

This book therefore is especially welcome as a sound guide for the teacher and the participant in exercising to music.

Whilst lecturing in the Physical Education and Sports Science Department at Loughborough University, I had the pleasure of working with the authors on their training programmes for teachers of exercise to music and I was able to observe their work at the Central YMCA at first hand. This book is in fact an extension of that work, based on solid experience and considerable expertise. It will certainly ensure that the ongoing development of exercise to music will now be along safe and professional lines.

Rex Hazeldine
Loughborough University of Technology

Introduction

In this book we hope to give to all of those who take part in 'Exercise to Music' classes guidelines by which they can judge the quality of the classes they attend. By 'exercise to music' we mean any exercise class that uses music as part of the class rather than just for background noise, be it 'aerobics', 'stretch', 'keep fit', 'conditioning', or any other title that may be temporarily fashionable. Throughout the book we have used 'she', although we assume that teachers and participants in classes will be both male and female.

Exercise to music has attracted many people who previously did not exercise. Some will have become bored with it, others put off by bad teaching. If taught well, however, exercise to music is an excellent and safe vehicle through which to obtain a general all-round fitness:

1 A good class will contain all of the components of physical fitness: cardio/vascular and respiratory fitness, muscular strength and endurance, flexibility and motor fitness.
2 A good class will be safe. It will have a warm-up and a cool-down, contain safe exercises and it will be related to the fitness levels of all the participants.
3 A good class will be progressive. It will teach the participants to monitor their progress and to learn about 'fitness'.
4 A good class will provide a variety of movement and provide opportunities to be creative and improve movement quality.
5 A good class will be enjoyable and not a fight against fatigue.
6 A good class will be satisfying and fulfilling; it will be a pleasurable, shared experience and not a competition.
7 A good class will be a social as well as a physical experience.

We believe that exercise can be of considerable benefit to everyone both physically and mentally and ought to be seen as a necessary ingredient in the daily life-style of people of all ages. Just as it can be fashionable to exercise, it can be equally fashionable to 'knock' exercise. Of course there is an element of risk, particularly if people are ill advised and badly taught. Driving a car may be risky; wearing a seat belt will reduce that risk. After reading this book we hope that, metaphorically, you will wear your seat belt secure in the knowledge that you are taking precautions, and convinced of the due value of the benefits of physical activity.

1

Examine Yourself

Can you identify yourself in the following:

1 Outwardly confident; matching leotard, tights, legwarmers, and head band; looking as though you are the last person on earth to need exercise.
2 Slightly overweight, nervous, and wearing the largest T shirt that money can buy to hide the odd bulge here and there.
3 Enthusiastic, serious, dedicated; able to drop the occasional phrase into the conversation which shows the depth of your knowledge – 'oh yes, my cardiovascular system has improved since I started classes'.
4 Fully dressed, observing, – having 'just come along with a friend', in your forties and admitting to 30; worried looking and wondering what on earth you are doing in the company of all of these 'youngsters'.
5 Male, not a games or racket player; an occasional jogger, embarrased that any of your friends should see you, in this female-dominated activity, doing 'aerobics'.
6 Unconcerned, uninformed, but knowing you are going to feel better having taken the class.

If you can see yourself in any one, or a combination, of the above, you deserve a round of applause. It is quite easy to poke fun at any stereotype, and some of the above are regarded as amusing stereotypes. Yet the most important thing is that you *are* included in the above; that you are making the effort; that you have not yet taken the easy, indolent, way out. It does not matter that you need or want to look attractive in your class, that you are slightly overweight now or that you are ill at ease when you first start. The confidence and benefits that regular exercise will give you, will make the effort worth while.

A great drawback for people taking classes in Exercise to Music, however, is that many are participating within an information vacuum; they have no yardstick by which they can identify or measure their progress towards their objectives. People start going to exercise classes for a variety of reasons and the whole experience can be socially enticing. Glossy magazines, the national press, television and the whole cosmetic and fashion industry contribute in the seduction. Perhaps, for some, physiological improvement may be a spur, but this is the exception rather than the rule. While it is easy to start a class, it may not be so easy to sustain an interest when some of the gloss has worn off. The capacity to identify or clarify your aims and objectives is vital as this extra knowledge helps to sustain interest by introducing the possibility of identifying real progress for yourself. To know how you can progress, to know why you are improving, and to be able to measure that improvement other than by a subjective feeling that you are 'getting fitter', can be overpoweringly important in turning a fad into a healthy long-lasting and gainful habit.

It is important to view your class in a positive way. You should see it as aiming to: improve general fitness, shape and poise; improve health, appearance and confidence; relax the body and mind; relax tension and reduce stress.

To see your class in these terms, however, and to be able to identify specific objectives for you as an individual, you must build up your knowledge of:

1 The qualities which a good teacher should possess and guidelines to teaching.
2 General fitness theories and a case for exercise.
3 Fitness testing.
4 Basic anatomy and physiology.
5 The structure of a class of Exercise to Music.
6 The use of music.
7 Exercise to music and its contribution to physical fitness at all levels.
8 Controversial exercises.
9 Safety concerns.
10 Potential injuries, their prevention and basic treatment.
11 Nutrition.

The following chapters will help you to do this.

2

Examine Your Teacher

Teacher does not always know best! Many problems, doubts and insecurities, which preoccupy members of a class are directly attributable to bad teachers, either through their lack of knowledge, lack of interest, lack of concern and lack of planning or foresight. Teachers cannot be all things to all students, but this should be their aim, and at least they ought to be many things to many students.

There are a number of ways in which you can judge your teacher and many clues if you know where to look. When you turn up for a class, are the facilities available for the class to start at the prescribed time? Have you been on a 'chase the caretaker', or 'hunt the light switch' escapade? Is a first aid box and a telephone available for emergencies?

Does the teacher present herself in an attractive way, in her physical appearance and manner? Are you made welcome? Good teachers will introduce themselves, giving you their name, experience, and qualifications, and inviting questions from you at the end of the session. A teacher should explain what the aims and purposes of the class are, and what she hopes all the class will achieve. If you are a new student, the teacher should speak to you individually before you start exercising in order to assess your capabilities, and to find out if there are any reasons why you should not exercise.

A good teacher will have all the necessary equipment for the class immediately available, and in working order. Mats for floorwork should be clean, appropriate and accessible. Her tapes and audio equipment should be suitable. Even at the back of the class, you should be able to hear the music quite clearly. One piece of music and routine should follow another, without a break for rewinding tapes, or finding the right tape. These sorts of problems can be greatly distracting and indicate a lack of organization in the teacher. If pulse rates are being taken and recorded, record sheets, pencils, and stopwatches should be available.

You should be encouraged by your teacher to wear comfortable clothing and appropriate footwear. This may sound like extremely elementary advice, and yet often it is never given. Restrictive clothing and inappropriate materials can be not only uncomfortable, but also unsafe. The habit of wearing plastic trousers during exercise can cause great discomfort and often distress because the plastic prevents the body's natural cooling mechanism from working as your body heat increases during exercise; dizziness and fainting can result.

Equally, performing aerobic exercise in bare feet or in the wrong sort of training shoes, can be a contributory factor to all sorts of injuries to the foot, ankles, calves, knees, shins, hips and back. Your foot is designed for two major functions; to help absorb the shock caused by impact with the ground, and to act as a rigid lever to help you walk. When exercising you will place a great deal more stress on your feet, particularly on the balls of the feet, than is normal. Barefoot exercise, therefore, is potentially very harmful: to wear appropriate footwear can significantly reduce the risk. Your exercise shoes need to give you support to arches and ankles. It should allow movement of the foot forwards, backwards and sideways, cushion your ankle, shins and lower back from the jarring on the balls of the feet caused by frequent repetition of jumping, hopping, skipping and running movements, and assist you in your posture. Running shoes, at one time thought to be the most suitable shoes on the market, are far from ideal as they are designed to protect against heelstrike, not impact by the ball of the foot. In addition, a thick, wide sole hampers safe lateral movements that often occur during exercise to music routines. In order to avoid problems you should wear a pair of shoes designed specifically for exercise to music.

To make the most of your class, you have to enjoy it, physically, emotionally and mentally. If you go home and suffer muscle soreness for days or feel emotionally drained and mentally deflated, your time has been wasted. A teacher, in her preparation of the music and exercises, in the assessment made of you and in general teaching method, is the single most important factor in determining the extent of your satisfaction or disillusionment with the exercise class. Essentially, a teacher has a class of individuals, not merely a class. In that class you should be made to feel like an individual, as well as a part of the class, and be taught as an individual as well as a part of the class.

DEMONSTRATION OF AN EXERCISE

As a student you should be shown the correct starting position for each exercise, and then given a clear demonstration with a brief verbal explanation. You should be allowed to join in the exercise as soon as possible, and be told what part of the body the exercise should be affecting and what good is being done, e.g. a correct sit-up is strengthening the stomach muscles. Students with bad backs, joint and muscle problems, ante- and postnatal and those with any ailments should be told to stop any exercise that causes pain.

CORRECTION OF EXERCISE

A good teacher will move around the class so that she can view you, the student, from all angles. This also gives you the opportunity of being near the teacher at some time during each class. Students should be reminded to breathe regularly and easily, and be encouraged to try to relax tense muscles.

The motor capabilities of students will vary significantly. A good teacher will be aware of these differences and will encourage students to work only within the limits of *their* ability. It is inadvisable to place someone physically in the correct position because there may be a very good physiological or anatomical reason for their inability to perform a particular task. Students should be encouraged verbally and by repeated and correct demonstration of the exercise to 'feel' the correct position.

Equally the fitness levels of students in a class differ significantly. Under physical stress, your ability to perform an exercise will deteriorate. A good teacher will be able to differentiate between failure due to motor capability or due to physical tiredness and react accordingly.

THE TEACHER'S VOICE Of the many factors which contribute to your enjoyment of an exercise class, the teacher's voice is of great importance. Clear, audible and precise words from a teacher can ensure that you understand the task in hand. A flexible and varied tone and pitch can create a lively and enjoyable rather than a dull atmosphere, can motivate or relax, and also help to give rhythm and tempo to your movement. Shouting is trying for both speaker and listener alike. The following phrases illustrate some of the correct words to use when teaching:

'Stretch as far as is comfortable.'
'Stop when you feel discomfort.'
'Reach as far as you are able.'
'Do as many as are comfortable.'
'Slowly and smoothly.'
'Keep a steady rhythm.'
'Bend your knees if necessary.'

Avoid at all costs a class where a teacher says:

'Bounce as far as you can.'
'Don't stop.'
'Go for the burn.'

In a class you should be made to feel comfortable and confident by the teacher. The size of your exercise area can be a problem which a thoughtful teacher will solve. In a small area, all of the available space should be used. Conversely you may feel exposed in a large area. All that is needed is for the area to be made smaller by using any available equipment, chairs, clothes, sports bags, etc.

A considerate teacher will set aside time at the end of the class when you can ask questions. There may be many aspects about which you are doubtful or curious. The more information you are given, the more secure you will feel and from this security will come confidence and enjoyment.

There are many clues available to help when you assess your teacher. If you can answer 'yes' to most of the following questions, you are in good hands:

Does your teacher know your name?
Are your achievements recognised with praise?
Have you been encouraged to communicate with your fellow students?
Are you encouraged by your teacher?
Are your exercises varied?
Does your teacher use new music?
Are any of the students asked to make up their own exercise sequence?
Is your class fun?
Are you learning about your body from the teacher?
Are you given any handouts related to exercise?

A student/teacher relationship is complex. A teacher can teach without being dictatorial; equally a student can learn without being made to feel inadequate, insecure, or ill-informed.

Fitness Theories

Everyone from physical educationalists, sports scientists, coaches and performers talk about it and everyone uses the word 'fitness'. Few, however, are able to explain what they mean by 'fitness'. It can mean different things to different people. When it is said that someone is 'looking fit', this is usually a reference to a general condition of apparent well-being, of looking good, which is often confused with being healthy. Being fit is not the same as being healthy, they are two quite separate conditions. A very fit athlete may not be healthy. Detailed medical examinations carried out on elite sportsmen and women have identified anaemia, hypertension, and even 'hole in the heart' cases. Conversely, non-athletes who were found to be quite healthy, were unable to swim or run for more than a few metres!

TOTAL FITNESS AND PHYSICAL FITNESS

1 Total fitness includes physical, nutritional, medical, mental, emotional and social fitness; and it can be described as the ability to meet the demands of the environment, plus a little in reserve for emergencies.
2 Physical fitness is only a part of total fitness; it is the capability of the heart, blood vessels, lungs and muscles to function at optimal efficiency. Physical fitness makes possible a life style that the physically unfit cannot enjoy. To develop and maintain physical fitness requires vigorous exercising of the whole body.

COMPONENTS OF PHYSICAL FITNESS

As someone involved in exercise to music classes, you should be able to answer the following questions.

1 What is physical fitness about?
2 What kind of exercise brings physical fitness?
3 How and how often should I exercise?

Physical fitness can be divided into five basic components: cardiovascular fitness, muscular strength, muscular endurance, flexibility and motor fitness.

Cardiovascular Fitness

Cardiovascular fitness is sometimes referred to as 'stamina' or 'endurance'. Other general terms used, and popularised in recent years by Dr K Cooper in his book *Aerobics*, are 'aerobic fitness' and 'aerobic power'. What all of these terms actually refer to is the efficiency of the heart and circulatory system, the workings of which can be described briefly as follows:

In order to work, muscles need oxygen which is carried in blood delivered to them by the arteries. If the work required of the muscles is increased progressively, as for example in a sensible graduated exercise to music programme, they will adapt to the extra work load by becoming more efficient in extracting oxygen from the same amount of blood. As this happens, the heart also adapts by beating at a slower, but more powerful rate.

The effect of these changes on the body's oxygen transport system is to make it more efficient and economic, enabling muscles to work harder for a longer period of time. In practical terms, the same exercise class becomes easier as the body adapts to the demands made upon it. This improvement in cardiovascular fitness is generally referred to as a 'training effect'. It is important here to note that, in spite of the fact that a class is called 'aerobic', it cannot be so unless it contains an aerobic content that lasts for approximately 20 minutes, during which time students are working at between 60% to 80% of their estimated maximum heart rate. More will be said about this in Chapter 5.

Muscular Strength

Muscular strength is the ability of a muscle to exert maximum force to overcome a resistance. By progressively increasing the amount of resistance a muscle must overcome, the muscle will be trained to work more efficiently. A weight trainer will become stronger by increasing the weight lifted and a student in an exercise to music class will become stronger by performing different exercises involving progressively greater resistance. For example, body weight may be used to provide greater resistance in attempting to increase arm strength.

1 Press-up against a wall.
2 Press-up on knees and hands.
3 Press-up on toes and hands.

Muscular strength is needed to counteract skeletal muscular strains and pulls as greater demands are made on the body.

Muscular Endurance

Muscular endurance is the ability of a muscle or a group of muscles to exert force to overcome a resistance for an extended period of time. This capability of the muscles to work continuously is developed in an exercise to music programme by performing a high number of repetitions of an exercise with a comparatively low resistance.

Flexibility

Flexibility refers to the capability of an individual to use the muscles and the skeletal joints throughout the full potential range of movement. Flexibility exercises involve lengthening the muscles, and are aimed directly at extending the range of movement of a

Press-up against a wall
Remember to keep the
stomach tight.

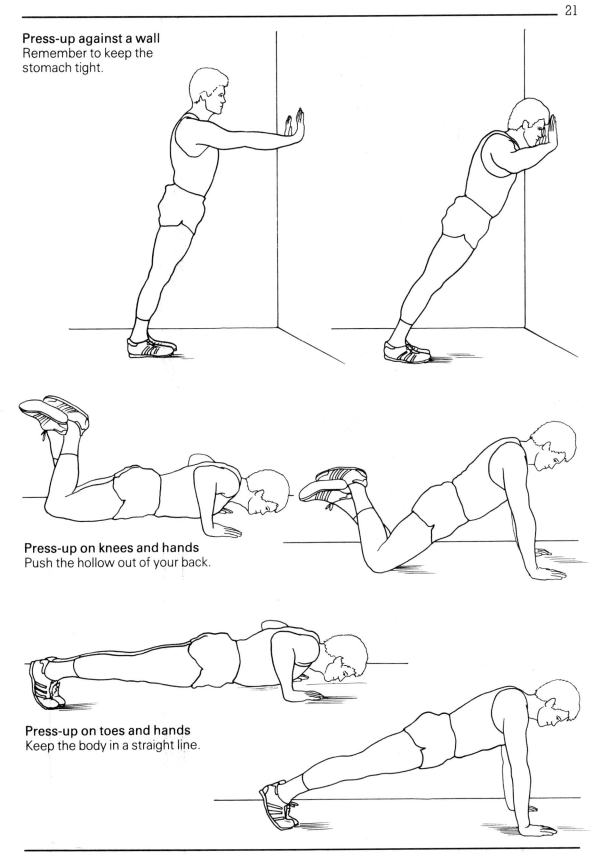

Press-up on knees and hands
Push the hollow out of your back.

Press-up on toes and hands
Keep the body in a straight line.

joint or muscle. The term 'stretching' has come to be accepted in describing these kinds of exercises, although technically the muscles are in fact relaxing. Flexibility exercises must be performed statically and progressively and only after the body has been warmed up.

Some people use the expression 'mobility', instead of 'flexibility'. In this book, however, mobility exercises refer to gentle, rhythmic movements taken only up to, but not beyond, the current range of movement of a joint or muscle, e.g. arm circling. This type of movement should be used as part of a warm-up in an exercise class to prepare the joints and muscles for exercise. It may also be called 'limbering up' or 'loosening up'.

Motor Fitness

Motor fitness refers to factors such as agility, balance, reaction time, co-ordination, power and speed. Some of these aspects are obviously inter-related but all have an important contribution to make towards physical fitness. Improvement of these factors will tend to allow movements to be performed more skilfully and thus you may achieve the same results with less expenditure of effort. In a class, for example, agility, balance and co-ordination may be improved by building on dance-type routines of gradually increasing difficulty. Power and speed, on the other hand, may be improved by varying the tempo and intensity of particular movements. Some aspects of motor fitness tend to be taught only indirectly, for example, co-ordination and balance, but their contribution to the 'quality' of movement is significant and should not be ignored. Balance refers to your ability to hold the centre of gravity of your body over a comparatively small base or basal area. The exact nature of this ability is highly complicated and the result of a co-ordination of action of the eyes, ears, neuromuscular system and control and tension of the muscles.

On a practical level, this has repercussions in an exercise to music class. Because balance is lost when you cannot maintain the centre of gravity over the base, it is better, if you are a beginner, to use a large base, and not to expect to be able to transfer weight in control between different balance positions. Conversely, a gymnast can be expected to transfer weight from one small base to another, whilst still retaining control. For example they can stand on one hand and transfer the weight on to their other hand without overbalancing or losing control. Your exercise to music class should include routines that explore balances and include gaining, maintaining and losing balance. They should also teach awareness of the body parts and their relation to one another during choreographed and co-ordinated movement routines. Eventually, even as a beginner, you may be able to regain poise after being thrown off balance.

As a student in exercise to music classes, you should aim to improve your performance in all five of the above components. It is quite possible, and in fact quite usual, to have a high score in one component and a low score in another. A good exercise to music class should include exercises aimed at improving each component, but, fortunately, capability in more than one component may be developed as a result of one particular exercise.

As you can now see, physical fitness is specific in that you are able to concentrate on one aspect to the exclusion of others. Bodybuilders, for example, will score very highly on the muscular strength component and look very 'fit' and 'healthy'. However, unless they take up something like jogging or cycling, they will score very poorly in any test of cardiovascular fitness. Similarly, runners may score very highly in cardiovascular tests, but ought not to neglect training schedules that improve the strength and flexibility for muscles of the arms, chest, back and abdomen. In a good exercise to music programme the opportunity is there for the student to obtain a high level of physical fitness in all components.

FACTORS AFFECTING PHYSICAL FITNESS

For everyone involved in exercise there are certain factors which have a significant effect on any attempt to improve physical fitness levels. Some factors can be influenced by the individual, others are hereditary in nature, and therefore beyond our influence.

Smoking

Smoking may contribute to premature death: it will certainly affect physical fitness levels whatever that level may be. When a smoker participates in a class of exercise to music performance efficiency is significantly impaired because a smoker's body does not use the oxygen available efficiently, and a smoker has a faster heart rate than would be necessary if that person did not smoke. Smokers should not comfort themselves by reference to fellow non-smoking class members, who may be less fit, and having more difficulty than themselves. They should compare potential physical fitness levels, and realise that while they smoke they will never realise their own potential. However, it is better for the smoker to take part in regular exercise classes, because these may help to minimise slightly the adverse physical effects of smoking. You should not smoke; if you do, you should exercise.

Nutrition and Diet

Nutrition and diet can affect your physical fitness. What you eat and when you eat will affect most components of physical fitness to differing degrees. Much more will be said in this context in Chapter 11. Suffice to say, that exercise makes extra demands upon the body's energy sources: if these are not replenished by a balanced diet, then the onset of fatigue during exercise will be brought forward. Under certain circumstances if, for example, an individual were on a very low calorie diet, there may be a constant feeling of fatigue or tiredness before, during and after exercise.

Sex Differences

Sex differences have to be considered by all of you who exercise and by teachers of exercise, but opinions differ about how much attention should be paid to this. In the past, levels of physical performance between males and females have been quite distinct. However, due to a greater understanding of the physiological differences between the sexes, better informed teachers, improved training methods and the raising of aspirations and goals, the gap between fitness and performance of men and women is closing all the time. When you exercise you ought to bear in mind the physiological differences between the sexes, particularly in respect of the flexibility, and muscular strength components, for example, women are in general more flexible in the joints than men: men are potentially stronger than women.

Body Type

Body type does have an effect on your response to exercise and should be kept in mind when you set out what you expect for yourself from your exercise programme. The structure of the body is more or less the same (bearing in mind the sex differences) in most individuals. However, body *types* do differ quite significantly and there is little that you can do to change your basic body type. Exercise and sensible eating will improve your shape and enable you to make the most of your body type, but neither will change that type.

There are three basic body types or somatotypes.

1 Ectomorphs: ECTOMORPHS are long and lean, with narrow shoulders and hips. They have very little fat or muscle bulk. Virtually all top-class long distance runners come from this type.

2 Mesomorphs: MESOMORPHS are broad shouldered, narrow waisted, and powerfully hipped; the classical triangular shape. Most top class sprinters and gymnasts come from this type.

3 Endomorphs: ENDOMORPHS tend to be short, with wide hips and of large proportions. They gain weight easily and, even when not overweight, tend to be rounded. Generally speaking, they do not excel athletically.

As we have said, all body shapes can be improved, but there is a limit to the extent of this improvement which has to be accepted by everyone who exercises, and has to be taken into account by all teachers of exercise. There is very little worse that a teacher can do than to give their students expectations of improvement in body shape which contradict basic somatotype and are therefore unrealisable regardless of the effort put into exercise by the student.

Hereditary

Hereditary characteristics determine, to a large extent, both the effect of exercise upon you, and your physical and movement ability. There is a constant and long-standing debate about the conflicting claim of hereditary and environment. A commonly held view at the present time is that physical ability is 75% genetic and 25% training and environment. Undoubtedly somatotype, as described above, is hereditary; it is inevitable that you will, to some extent, inherit your parents body type characteristics.

You should not be despondent, however, because you are not a highly skilled mesomorph. In an imperfect world there are a few who realise their full potential. Consequently an indolent, sedentary, well fed mesomorph may look more like an endomorph, than a well motivated, well exercised and sensibly eating 'natural' endomorph. You have no excuse, therefore, to throw away your training shoes, put on your slippers, and relax in front of the TV until inactivity sets in permanently.

Age

Age is often thought of as a barrier to exercise. Of course a younger person will be more capable of achieving a higher level of fitness than someone over fifty years of age; but don't reach for those slippers or that TV switch just yet. Age is not a barrier to exercise, it is merely one factor amongst many that you and your teacher should consider.

There are many elderly people who today are virtually housebound as a result of well-intentioned but misguided concern and advice. The custom that encourages them to 'put-up their feet and let the young ones do the fetching and carrying', is misguided both practically and physiologically. Inactivity in the elderly leads to inability to be active. Muscles that are not used atrophy, joints that remain immobile, stiffen and become restricted in movement. Correct exercise can be a rejuvenator.

Pregnancy

For women who are pregnant, regular exercise does not have to cease. However, there are many changes that occur in the body due to hormonal adjustment and consideration must be given to this regarding jogging, stretching and certain muscle exercises (e.g. abdominals). It is unwise to stress yourself; as the pregnancy advances restrictions on your capability to exercise will increase and, therefore, you must ensure that you always 'listen to your body' and learn from available sources (e.g. antenatal classes). The postnatal period is again very individual but you must remember that hormone levels will only gradually return to normal. Some research shows significant presence of 'pregnancy' hormones up to 5 months after the birth so extreme care must be taken during your return to normal exercise sessions.

Physical fitness, its components, and the factors that affect it, should now be an open book to you. But to stop there, and to assume that physical fitness is an end in itself, may be a prescription for temporary narcissism and obsession. Your expectation of your exercise class should be far greater.

TOTAL FITNESS

Total fitness should be your aim and is a far higher ideal than any of its parts. It is a state of being rather than doing, and available to all of you regardless of skill level, movement quality, somatotype, sex, or any other hereditary or environmental influence. Possessing total fitness results in feeling well and looking good, and enables you to live, rather than exist in our western culture with all of the pressures and problems associated with it.

In the early years of Physical Training in schools, when a zombie-like adherence to straight lines in class, and repetitive vaulting over boxes was seen as the panacea of all ills, social and physical; physical fitness was made an end in itself. Physical education classes changed this idea to some extent, by trying to educate through the physical, extending the range of activities but concentrating on skill related fitness. The concept of total fitness, with health related fitness as a part of it, was given scant regard.

If total fitness is your aim, you have to develop an independence of attitude that makes you self-reliant; you will exercise because you value fitness, not because you are told to exercise. The information in this book, will, we hope help you achieve this aim. If you refer back to the beginning of this chapter, you will see that total fitness includes physical, nutritional, medical, mental, emotional and social fitness. We have already explained physical fitness, its components, and the factors that affect it. Nutritional fitness will be dealt with in Chapter 11.

HOW EXERCISE CONTRIBUTES TO HEALTH AND WELL-BEING

Recent relevant scientific evidence leads to the conclusion that the less active members of the general public would benefit from increasing their levels of physical activity. The psychological benefits which have been observed in controlled studies include increases in extroversion, self-confidence, self-awareness, and improvements in recall in the elderly. Many of you who exercise will know the intense feeling of well-being that follows a good exercise to music class. This mental and emotional stimulation may lead to a social confidence which surprises all who know you. Provided that exercise levels are increased gradually, harmful effects are extremely unlikely.

As a result of exercise there are marked physiological improvements in the normal functions of many body systems. Conversely, inactivity leads to a deterioration in body functions and a decline in physical ability.

Obesity is associated with heart disease and diabetes. In the past, weight reduction has depended almost exclusively upon dietary control or the prescription of appetite depressant drugs. Recent successful investigations in this field, which have included exercise as well as dietary control, indicate that exercise must be considered to be as important as dietary restriction in the treatment of obesity. If you are a beginner in an exercise to music class and take part three times a week, your increased expenditure of energy may result in a significant weight loss. Perhaps of greater significance is the recent demonstration that exercise has a stimulating effect on metabolism which persists throughout the day, varies the metabolic rate and leads to the loss of appreciably more fat than would have been predicted for the exercise undertaken. The increase in energy expenditure due to regular moderate exercise does not appear to be accompanied by a compensatory increase in appetite and energy intake. The biochemistry of the obese diabetic is also improved by regimes which include regular physical activity.

There is evidence to suggest that there is a low incidence of coronary heart disease amongst those who are involved in high levels of physical activity. A recent investigation of British middle-aged male civil servants in sedentary jobs found that those taking vigorous exercise during their lifetime suffered a heart attack with only one third the frequency of matched controls who were inactive. In a study of dockers in San Francisco who were followed for 22 years, men classified as being in jobs requiring repeated outbursts of high energy output had a death rate from coronary heart disease only half that of the men in jobs requiring a medium or low energy output. The level of 'high output energy' was high compared to that common in the general population.

For many patients with cardiac disease, angina limits their tolerance to exercise. Angina occurs when the oxygen demand of a part of the muscles of the heart (myocardium) exceeds the supply, usually because the coronary blood flow is impeded by a partial blocking (atheroma) of the coronary arteries.

The oxygen demand of the heart muscle depends mainly upon individual heart rate and blood pressure. As the effect of training is to lower the heart rate, this in turn also leads to a reduction in the myocardial oxygen demand: symptoms of angina therefore occur only at a greater level of physical exertion.

Many of the worthwhile benefits of rehabilitation and exercise training for patients convalescing from myocardial infarction (heart attack) are psychological and arise from rebuilding the patient's confidence in his ability to take exercise without harm. (In addition, it is possible that exercise may reduce the rate of recurrent infarction (attacks) in these patients, but, so far, there is little evidence of this in controlled trials).

Those who are disabled by chronic respiratory disease can improve their performance up to the limits set by their disease and thus may cope with their daily tasks more successfully. Similarly, with chronic muscle diseases, determined efforts to get the best of the remaining muscles by training can achieve a worthwhile extension of independent mobility.

It is clear that exercise can be of considerable benefit to everyone, physically, psychologically, emotionally and socially, and may be seen by you as a part of your lifestyle for the whole of your life. It is not enough to take part in an exercise to music class for a short time, and be dependent upon your teacher for motivation. The knowledge you are gaining from this book should be digested so that you can take your own informed decisions about exercise. This may mean that you swim, jog, weight train or circuit train, as well as exercise to music. The important thing is that you accept the fact that exercise is essential to you.

Fitness Testing

In order to attain an independence of decision in respect of your exercise requirements, or to judge the effectiveness of your exercise to music class in fulfilling the components of physical fitness, you ought to be able to measure or test your fitness. Fitness testing can vary in accuracy and sophistication, depending upon your requirements.

Sometimes all you need is a personal comparative measure, for, after all, exercise to music should not be competitive. General self-evaluation can be useful. When you first start exercising, you may not be able to carry on a conversation when the tempo of exercise increases. After a few weeks, this may be possible; an obvious improvement. Equally, you may, and should, find that you are coping with the class much more easily as you become a regular attender; breathlessness decreases, you are less flushed, deadness of the legs is no longer apparent, your desire or need to stop lessens, and at the end of a class you feel capable of continuing.

There are some generally reliable, specific, tests for cardiovascular, muscular strength, muscular endurance and flexibility fitness, which you can do for yourself. You can also compare your performance with sets of 'norms' which have been devised as a result of testing literally thousands of individuals.

1 a Specific self-evaluation of a non-sophisticated nature of your cardiovascular system can be achieved by heart-rate monitoring. If you take your heart rate within the first twenty seconds after exercise, it will give a good indicator of the level at which you are exercising. To do this, you must find the pulse, in the wrist, or the neck, and count the number of beats in a fifteen second time span. If you multiply this number by 4, you will find your heart rate for one minute, which should then be referred to one of the columns of 'target heart rate', as shown in chart, opposite and you will know at what rate you are exercising.

NOTE: the maximum heart rate is estimated by taking your age away from 220. A target heart rate which would ensure a 'training gain' would be at least 60%, or at the most 85%, of your maximum heart rate. When you first enter a fitness programme, your target heart rate, during exercise, should be 60% of the predicted maximum heart rate. After adequate progression and time, your target heart rate can be increased to as much as 85% of the predicted maximum heart rate. You should remember, however, that the heart rate decreases with age, and therefore your target and maximum heart rate will also decrease as you get older.

Age	Maximum heart rate	Target heart rate		
		60%	70%	85%
20–29	200–191	120–114	140–134	170–162
30–39	191–181	114–109	133–127	161–154
40–49	180–171	108–103	126–120	153–145
50–59	170–161	102– 97	119–113	144–137

b A second, and simple way, of assessing an improvement in your cardiovascular fitness is by means of a one-minute shuttle run.

One-minute Shuttle run

1 Place two markers, A and B, 9 metres apart.
2 Sit down for 10 minutes, and then take and record your pre-exercise heart rate for 15 seconds.
3 Commence your shuttle run; running from A to B and back to A counting as one repetition. Complete seven repetitions in one minute, at approximately eight seconds for each repetition.
4 Sit down immediately, and take and record your exercise heart rate for 15 seconds.
5 Remain seated and take and record your heart rate six more times, at intervals of fifteen seconds, which we will call your post-exercise heart rates.

You should record your results on a chart as follows:

Heart Rate Record Table

DATE	25.12.85			
Pre-Exercise Heart Rate	20			
Exercise Heart Rate	35			
1 Post-Exercise Heart Rate	30			
2 Post-Exercise Heart Rate	26			
3 Post-Exercise Heart Rate	24			
4 Post-Exercise Heart Rate	22			
5 Post-Exercise Heart Rate	22			
6 Post-Exercise Heart Rate	21			

If you complete the above test after spending some time attending your exercise to music classes you will have some indication of improvements in your cardiovascular system, for example:

a Your pre-exercise heart rate may decrease.
b Your exercise heart rate may decrease.
c The rate at which your post-exercise heart rate returns to the same level as your pre-exercise heart rate may increase. In other words, it may be that your post exercise heart rate, number 4, will be the same as your pre-exercise heart rate.

NB: If you have not exercised for some time, you should refer to Chapter 8, before taking the above test.

2

Specific self-evaluation of a non-sophisticated nature of your muscular strength and endurance may be obtained from a one-minute sit-up test, or a press-up test.

We have combined these two components because it is extremely difficult, particularly without equipment, to identify exercises which can isolate from each other the muscular strength or muscular endurance element, let alone to measure each element. Yet again motivation can be critical in these tests, as can be the controlling of the technique used. Nevertheless, both of these tests are generally representative, and may be compared to 'norms'.

Test 1 – One-minute Timed Sit-up

1 You should lie face up on a mat on the floor, knees bent at right angles, or heels about 50 cm from the buttocks, with hands either side of the head. A partner should hold your ankles firmly for support. (See below.)
2 At a 'go' signal from your partner you then perform as many correct sit-ups as you can within a one minute period. Your elbows should touch alternately the opposite knee as you come into the 'up' position. Your partner should take the count.
3 After each sit-up you should return to the lying position, before going up again. Your shoulders must be returned to touch the mat, but the head need not touch. (See below.)
4 Your score is determined by counting the number of completed sit-ups in one minute, and compared to the norms below.

NB: You should breathe easily during the exercise and not hold your breath.

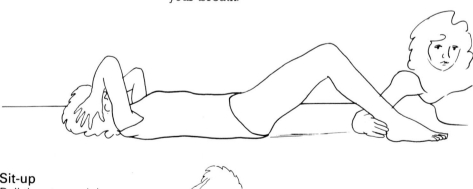

Sit-up
Pull the stomach in.

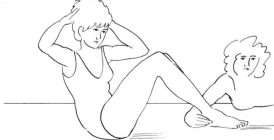

Sit-up Test Score

| Age | Female | | | | |
---	Exc	Good	Ave	Fair	Poor
Under 35	39	34	25	16	10
36–45	39	29	18	10	4
46+	24	20	14	8	2

| Age | Male | | | | |
---	Exc	Good	Ave	Fair	Poor
Under 35	45	41	33	24	18
36–45	42	38	27	19	11
46+	38	33	21	16	10

Test 2 – Press-up

1 You should take up the appropriate positions as shown below depending upon whether you are a man or woman.
2 You perform as many correct press-ups as possible, ensuring that your chin touches the floor each time before your arms are straightened, your body should remain in a straight line from heels or knees to shoulders.

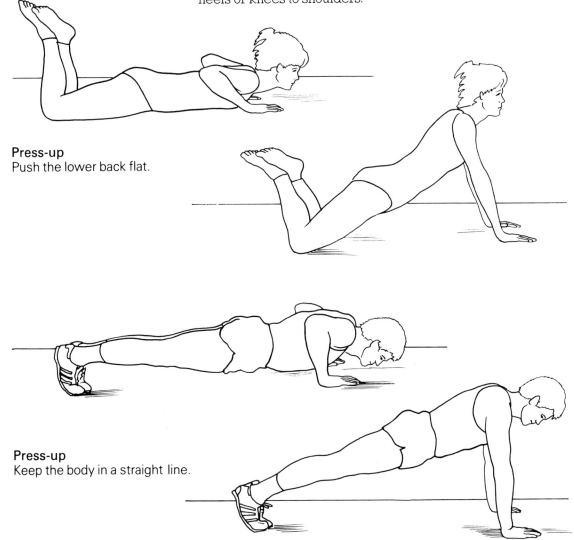

Press-up
Push the lower back flat.

Press-up
Keep the body in a straight line.

3 Your score is determined by counting the number of completed press-ups. You may stop and start again during this test, but you must not leave the press-up position once you have assumed it. You may compare your score to the norms below.

Press-up Test Score

	Female (b)				
Age	Exc	Good	Ave	Fair	Poor
Under 35	40	33	25	14	5
36–45	35	30	19	10	3
46+	30	23	14	6	1

(b) – Modified press-up.

	Male				
Age	Exc	Good	Ave	Fair	Poor
Under 35	45	40	30	20	12
36–45	40	35	26	21	9
46+	36	30	20	10	5

3

Specific self-evaluation of a non-sophisticated nature of your flexibility can be obtained from a simple trunk flexion, or sit and reach test.

As flexibility is specific to one particular joint, there is no simple, general flexibility test of total body flexibility. However, trunk flexion has proved to be as reliable an indicator as any.

In order to measure your performance, you need a tape measure, two pieces of sticky tape, and a flat, thin board, approximately 1 metre long by 50 cm wide. The tape measure and tape are arranged on the board as shown below.

a The board is placed on the floor.
b The tape measure is placed on the board, and secured in place by means of one of the pieces of sticky tape.
c The second piece of sticky tape is placed at right angles to the tape measure, at the 38 cm mark.

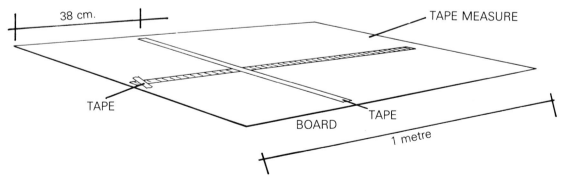

Test 3 – Flexibility

1 Do a short warm-up including stretching exercises prior to this test, particularly of hamstrings and lower back, with no bouncing or jerky movements.

2 Remove shoes.

3 Sit and place your heels at the taped line which crosses the 38 cm mark, about 25 cm to 30 cm apart.

4 Exhale, and slowly reach forward with both hands, one directly on top of the other, as far as possible to touch the tape measure, holding this position for 3 seconds. Be sure that you do not bend the knees, bounce or jerk, or lead with one hand.

5 Your score is determined by counting the most distant point, in centimetres, reached by your finger tips on the tape measure. The best of three attempts should be recorded and compared to the scores below.

Flexibility Test Score in cms

| Age | Female | | | | |
	Exc	Good	Ave	Fair	Poor
Under 35	58	53	46	35	28
36–45	58	53	43	30	25
46+	56	48	38	28	23

| Age | Male | | | | |
	Exc	Good	Ave	Fair	Poor
Under 35	53	48	38	25	18
36–45	56	48	35	28	13
46+	51	43	33	23	13

With the above suggestions you can get some general idea of how fit you are when you first start exercising and you should be able to measure any improvement after you have been exercising for a period of time. Of course, none of these tests are of a sophisticated nature, and they are fitness tests *not* medical tests indicating whether or not you are in good or bad health.

There are more sophisticated tests which you can take to test both your fitness level and your state of health. These may involve sphygnomanometers, bicycle ergometers, computer-based gas analysers, electrocardiographs, X-rays, etc, but are usually quite expensive, and need a qualified sports scientist or doctor to interpret the results.

Basic Anatomy and Physiology

Before you can begin to assess your exercise to music class, it is essential to understand how the body works.

THE SKELETON

VERTEBRAL COLUMN OR BACKBONE

The vertebral column is made up of 33 vertebrae which subdivide into the following groups:

7 cervical vertebrae (neck)
12 thoracic vertebrae (dorsal)
5 lumber vertebrae (loin)
5 sacral vertebrae (rump)
4 coccygeal vertebrae (tail)

The 5 vertebrae in the sacral area are fused to form the sacrum. The 4 vertebrae in the coccygeal area are fused to form the coccyx.

THORAX

The thorax is a dome shaped structure. It is made up of:
Sternum or breastbone
12 pairs of ribs
12 thoracic vertebrae.

THE PECTORAL OR SHOULDER GIRDLE

The pectoral girdle consists of:
2 Scapulae or shoulder blades
2 Clavicles or collar bones

The pectoral girdle provides a strong, mobile base for the attachment of the arms to the trunk. It is not adapted for weight bearing but for the performance of complex movements rather than simple movements.

THE PELVIC OR HIP GIRDLE

The pelvic girdle is made up of:
Ilium
Ischium
Pubis
Pubis Symphysis

The main function of the pelvic girdle is to provide a solid base through which weight can be transmitted to the lower limbs from the upper part of the body. It also provides the attachment for the powerful muscles of the leg and lower back.

UPPER LIMBS OR ARMS	These are made up of: Humerus or upper arm Radius and Ulna or lower arm 8 Carpals, 5 Metacarpals and 14 Phalanges form the hand
LOWER LIMBS OR LEGS	These are made up of: Femur or thigh bone Tibia or shin bone Fibula Patela or kneecap 7 Tarsals, 5 Metatarsals and 14 Phalanges form the foot
CRANIUM OR SKULL	Made up of a number of interlinking bone segments which fuse together gradually during the first few years of life to form a solid protective dome around the brain.

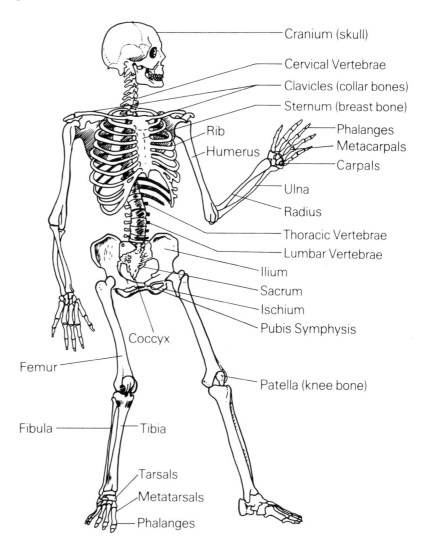

The Skeleton

Functions of the Skeleton

1 Protection: the skull protects the brain, the thorax protects the ribs, heart and lungs, the vertebral column protects the spinal cord and the pelvis protects the abdominal organs.

2 The marrow of the long bones constantly produces the red and white blood cells. This is an essential function when one considers that approximately 18 million cells die every minute. After a blood donor has given 440 cc of blood it takes three to four weeks for the body to restore the number of red cells that have been lost, although the white cells are replaced in a few hours.

3 Affords muscle attachments.

4 Allows movement through muscles working across joints.

5 Stores calcium and phosphorus, which are essential for growth and good health.

6 Gives the body its characteristic shape.

Bone

At birth, bones are made of cartilage. As a child grows, calcium is laid down and the cartilage gradually becomes bone. Developed bones have a compact outer layer and a honeycomb-like inner network.

Bone can be subdivided into the following types:

a Long bones: for example, femur and humerus which act as levers.

b Short bones: for example, carpals and tarsals which have relatively restricted movement while still allowing flexibility.

c Flat bones: for example, pelvis and scapulae which are both protective and allow for very strong muscle attachments for the major muscle groups.

d Irregular bones: for example, vertebrae.

JOINTS AND THEIR STRUCTURE

A joint occurs when a bone meets a bone.

There are three basic types of joint:

1 Immovable Joints: where bones are joined by cartilage or a system of dove-tailed edges, for example, the Skull.

2 Slightly Movable Joints: where two bony surfaces are united by ligaments alone, or ligaments with a fibrous cartilage interposed between the body surfaces, for example, the Vertebral Column.

3 Freely Movable Joints: where the ends of the bones are covered with cartilage and connected by a fibrous capsule which has a synovial membrane secreting fluid to lubricate the joints.

There are six types of freely movable joints:

a Gliding, where movement is over flat surfaces, for example, the Carpals and Tarsals.

b Hinge, where movement is in one plane only, for example, the elbow and knee. (See diagrams opposite.)

c Pivot, where movement is purely rotational, for example, in the neck, the Atlas and Axis.

d Condyloid, where the condyle fits into a concave surface allowing flexion and extension, for example, the head of the humerus and the clavicle.

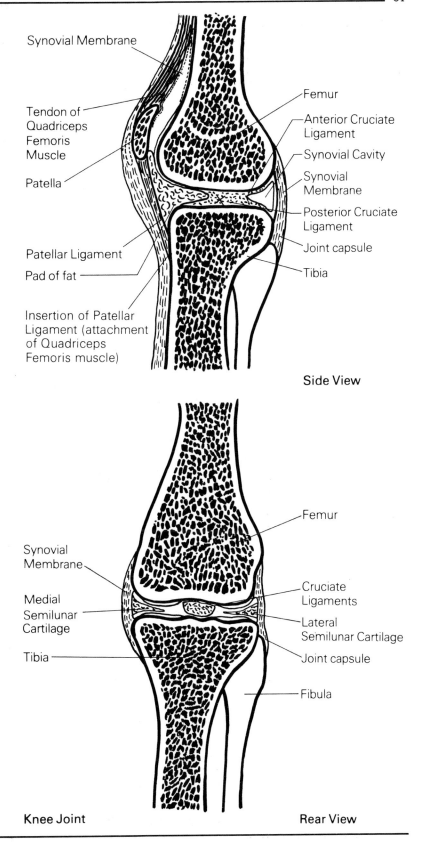

Synovial Membrane

Tendon of Quadriceps Femoris Muscle

Patella

Femur

Anterior Cruciate Ligament

Synovial Cavity

Synovial Membrane

Posterior Cruciate Ligament

Joint capsule

Patellar Ligament

Pad of fat

Tibia

Insertion of Patellar Ligament (attachment of Quadriceps Femoris muscle)

Side View

Synovial Membrane

Medial Semilunar Cartilage

Tibia

Femur

Cruciate Ligaments

Lateral Semilunar Cartilage

Joint capsule

Fibula

Knee Joint

Rear View

e Saddle, which is similar to Condyloid but the surfaces are concave and convex, for example, the base of the thumb.

f Ball and Socket, where a spherical head fits into a cup-like socket, allowing movement in all directions, for example, the shoulder joint and hip joint. (See diagrams below and right.)

Your capacity to perform movements in a class is limited by the structure of your joints. Some movements are impossible for you, and everyone else; other movements may be difficult to perform at the moment, but after correct instruction and practice this should not be the case.

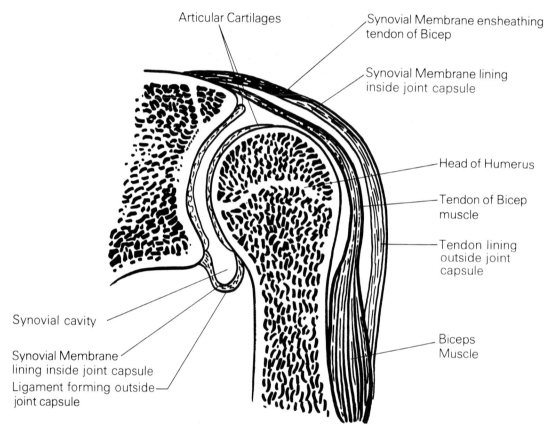

Articular Cartilages

Synovial Membrane ensheathing tendon of Bicep

Synovial Membrane lining inside joint capsule

Head of Humerus

Tendon of Bicep muscle

Tendon lining outside joint capsule

Synovial cavity

Synovial Membrane lining inside joint capsule

Ligament forming outside joint capsule

Biceps Muscle

Shoulder Joint

Cartilage

Cartilage, or gristle, is a glassy-looking, elastic tissue that helps to keep the joints together. It acts often as a shock absorber, for example, the semilunar cartilages in the knees, and the intervertebral discs.

Tissues Involved in Movement

a Tendons are non-elastic tissue bundles that connect muscles to bone. A muscle produces movement when it contracts.

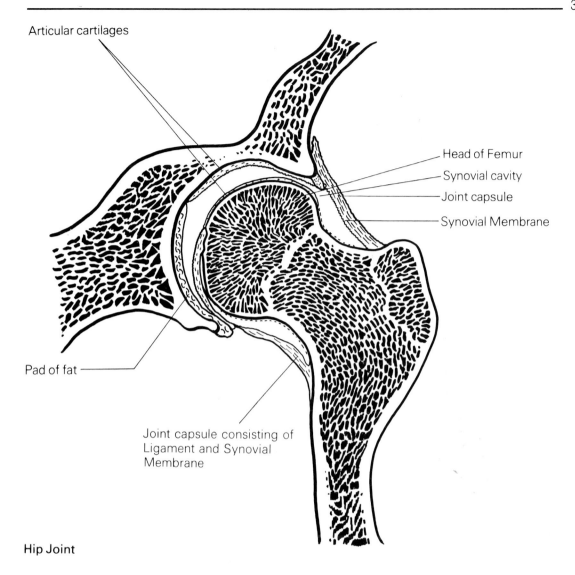

Articular cartilages

Head of Femur

Synovial cavity

Joint capsule

Synovial Membrane

Pad of fat

Joint capsule consisting of
Ligament and Synovial
Membrane

Hip Joint

b Ligaments are fibrous bands of tissue that usually connect the bones that form a joint. They support and stabilise the joints and help to prevent dislocation. Some ligaments, such as those on the vertebral column, cross and connect several joints. A ligamental sprain occurs when a ligament is overstretched and can be very serious if the ligament is completely torn or ruptured.

The Curvature of the Spine

The spine has to be very strong as it sustains the weight of the upper body and has to absorb force and shock. Its curvature, in four parts, has 400 muscles and scores of ligaments which hold it erect in place. This enables it to fulfill its function. Its inbuilt resistance takes all the strain when landing on the feet. If the spine was a straight column, it would have only approximately a sixteenth of its strength, and the brain would be severely damaged whenever the feet were placed down forcefully. The spine's shock absorbers, in the form of discs, move in relation to each other and also allow bending forwards, backwards and sideways.

The spine has its limitations both in terms of shock absorption and mobility: when it is overtaxed back trouble will result.

MUSCLES

Your capacity to move correctly and efficiently, sustain movement and exercise in general is also limited by the type, strength and bulk of your muscles.

Muscles and How They Work

Muscle tissue has the power to contract when it receives stimulation from the nerves. Of the three types of muscle, voluntary, involuntary and cardiac, we are particularly concerned with the first which is also known as the striated, striped or skeletal muscle.

Voluntary Muscles

Voluntary muscles make up the majority of the flesh of human beings. There are approximately 650 muscles in the body, which make up 35% to 40% of the total body weight. A striated/striped muscle fibre (see opposite), is a long thin tube consisting of an inner sarcoplasm with a surrounding wall of sarcolemna. Within this wall lie a number of nuclei. The sarcoplasm contains long contractile fibrils which consist of alternate segments, or granules, of light and dark material, which give the fibre a striped appearance.

Muscles are always in a state of *tone* or slight tension ready to react to a stimulus from their nerve supplies. Without this tone the body would collapse in a heap unable to hold its normal upright posture. When a stimulus occurs requiring contraction, the muscle fibres work on an *all or none* basis, either contracting completely or not at all. The strength of the contraction will depend upon the number of fibres brought into use. When stimulated, a muscle will need oxygen (O_2) and fuel to produce the necessary energy for the work it is to perform. This fuel is mainly in the form of glucose, which the muscle stores, and fats, which are sent via the blood. The muscle burns the substances by combining them with oxygen from the blood, water and carbon dioxide (CO_2) being produced as waste products. The chemical energy released in this process is used to form a bond between a phosphate and a substance called ADP, Adenosine Diphosphate. A further substance ATP, Adenosine Triphosphate, is formed in the same process. When a muscle performs work the ATP changes into ADP, producing energy. This is then used in the contraction of muscle fibres. Muscles working hard use a great deal of ATP and therefore need a great deal of fuel and oxygen to produce it. This is the reason why strenuous exercise demands large amounts of oxygen and causes deep and rapid breathing.

On the whole this is an inefficient system because approximately 25% of the energy is used to contract the muscle, and 75% is converted to heat and so lost; hence strenuous work makes you warm. Often when a muscle contracts, successive impulses pass to it and a continuous contraction occurs. After prolonged stimulation the contractions become slower and weaker and the muscle becomes fatigued because the carbohydrates are only partially broken down and cause a build-up of a harmful substance called lactic acid.

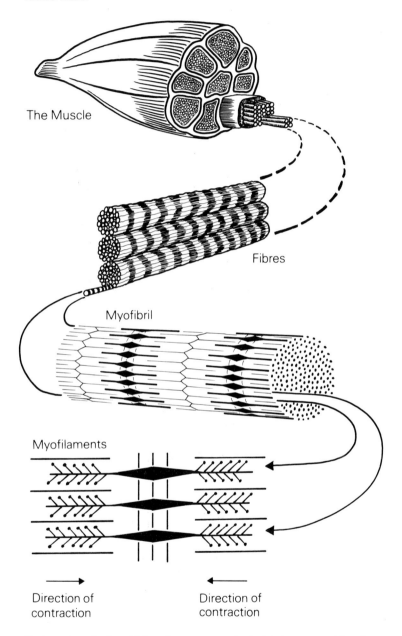

The Muscle

Fibres

Myofibril

Myofilaments

Direction of contraction

Direction of contraction

Striated or Striped Muscle – successively higher magnification

Movement Brought About by Muscle Action

Muscles bring about movement by way of their attachment to bones or cartilage, which act as levers. Muscle itself is liable to tear and is therefore attached by connective tissue forming tendons which merge with the muscle fibres and make a strong bond with the bones. Each attachment has an origin (fixed), and an insertion (movable), and muscles usually pull the two attachment points towards the centre. When a muscle contracts the fibres shorten and pull on the bones causing them to move together around a joint; the bones act as levers and the joints as a fulcrum.

The following terms are used to describe the various ways muscles work:

Flexion	to reduce the angle at the joint, or to bend a limb.
Extension	to return from flexion or increase the angle at the joint, or to straighten a limb.
Adduction	to bring towards the midline of the body.
Abduction	to take away from the midline of the body.
Elevation	to raise, as in lifting the shoulders.
Depression	to pull down, as in pulling down the shoulders.
Lateral Flexion	to bend sideways with the trunk or neck.
Rotation	rotary movement, inward or outward, about the long axis of the bone.
Circumduction	to circle part of the body, possible in the shoulder joint and hip joint.

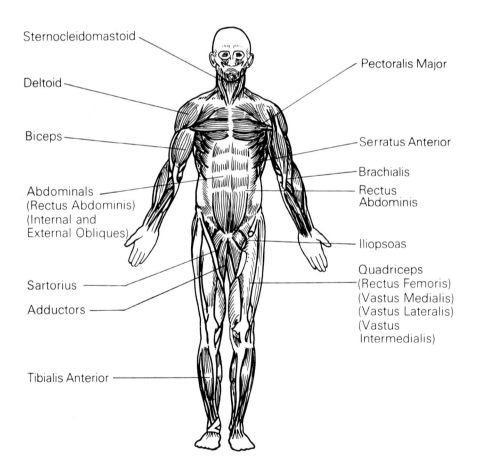

Sternocleidomastoid

Deltoid

Biceps

Abdominals
(Rectus Abdominis)
(Internal and
External Obliques)

Sartorius

Adductors

Tibialis Anterior

Pectoralis Major

Serratus Anterior

Brachialis

Rectus
Abdominis

Iliopsoas

Quadriceps
(Rectus Femoris)
(Vastus Medialis)
(Vastus Lateralis)
(Vastus
Intermedialis)

Muscle Chart Front

Most muscles work in *groups* rather than individually, acting in the following ways:

a *As the Prime Mover* – the muscle principally responsible for movement taking place.
b *As the Antagonist* – the muscle responsible for opposite movement which relaxes as the Prime Mover works.
c *As the Synergist* – the muscle which contracts to check unnecessary movement at the joints.
d *As the Fixator* – the muscle responsible for fixing the upper attachment.

It is not necessary for you to know every muscle in the body. It is useful, however, to know the major muscle groups and to understand their primary functions (see diagrams below and left). This can be worked out if you know the attachment points and joint(s) which is (are) crossed. This knowledge will help you understand the exercise to music schedules related to increasing strength, stamina and mobility.

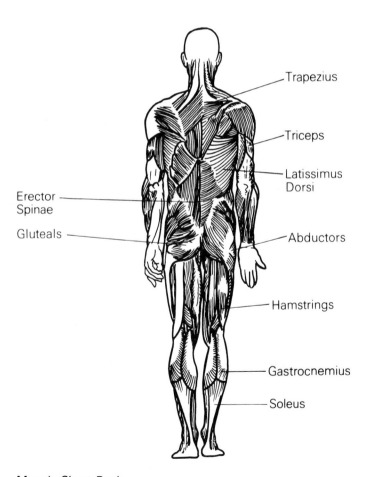

Muscle Chart Back

Elbow Extended

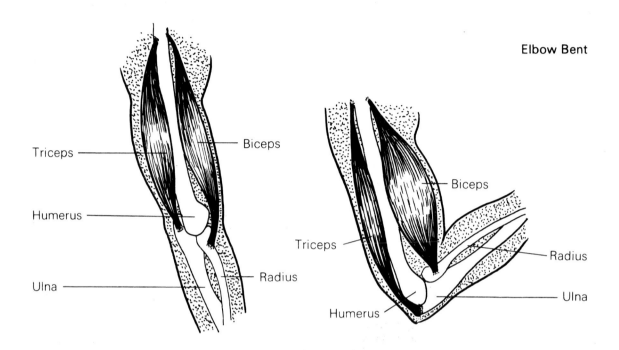

Triceps — Biceps

Humerus — Radius

Ulna —

Elbow Bent

Biceps —

Triceps — Radius

Humerus — Ulna

MUSCLE WORK

Muscles or groups of muscles are classified according to whether when they contract they shorten, lengthen or hold a fixed position.

1 *Concentric Contraction* occurs when a muscle shortens against resistance: for example, in elbow flexion the brachialis and biceps shorten bringing the forearm towards the upper arm.
2 *Eccentric Contraction* occurs when a muscle returns to its normal length after lengthening against resistance: for example, a tricep press in a seated position.
3 *Static Contraction* occurs when a muscle is actively engaged in holding a static position: for example, when stopping half way up from a knee bend.

Muscles need to be kept in constant use if they are not to lose condition. If muscles are not used their capacity for work is reduced, they become weaker, but do not lose the ability to grow stronger if exercised again.

When a heavier than normal demand is placed upon the muscles, they are stimulated into growing stronger. Such a resistance stresses the muscles and they adapt to accommodate the greater workload. As long as that load intensity remains constant, the muscle strength level will not improve any further. If the resistance at this stage is increased slightly, then the muscle will again get stronger. This is *progressive resistance training* with the muscle trying to stay one step ahead of the load by becoming stronger with each increased demand upon it.

Resistance exercises in your class offer a number of benefits including:

1 An improvement of tone in the muscle.
2 An improvement of skill. The more 'finely tuned' muscular response, resulting from the taking up of slack muscle, facilitates more accurate movement patterns and hence more efficient skill acquisition.
3 A better preparation for future demands. The well developed, strong and flexible body will be better able to cope with the physical demands that may be made upon it, either through work or exercise. The risk of poor posture or muscle and joint injury, which exists where there is a strength imbalance between reciprocal muscle groups, will be greatly reduced. This positive aspect can be eroded or reversed if training programmes are not of a balanced nature, for example, where there is a relative overdevelopment of a muscle, compared to its antagonist.
4 Improvement of self-confidence. An often underestimated aspect of strength development is the effect it has on an individual's self-confidence. Seeing evidence of improvement, both in shape or size and strength, leads to a sense of accomplishment which in turn reinforces self-belief and the ability to give commitment, a benefit which is often transferred to other aspects of daily life.

THE CIRCULATORY SYSTEM

Problems with your Circulatory System not only impair your ability to exercise safely, they can also severely impair your health.

The Circulatory System transports blood through the body which carries:

Oxygen	from the lungs to the body tissue.
Carbon Dioxide	from the cells to the lungs for elimination.
Nutrients	from the intestines and the liver, for example, glucose to the muscles and proteins for cell building.
Waste products	from the tissue, mostly to the kidneys.
Protective white cells and antibodies Hormones Drugs/Medicine and Heat	throughout the body.

The system performs a complete circuit through Arteries, Arterioles, Capillaries, Venules, Veins, and back to Arteries again. The blood is pumped through the system by the heart.

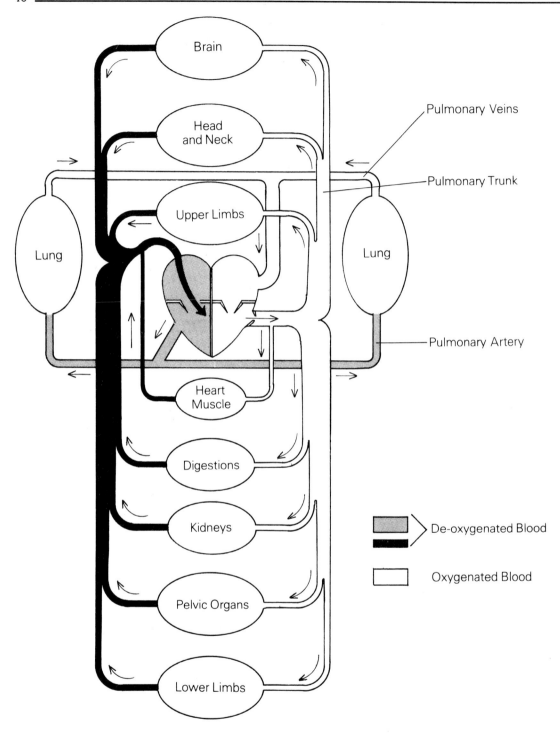

Cardiovascular System General Scheme of Circulation

The Heart

The heart is situated in the chest between the sternum and the spine. It has four chambers:

Right Atrium receives deoxygenated blood from the body.
Right Ventricle pumps deoxygenated blood to the lungs.
Left Atrium receives oxygenated blood from the lungs.
Left Ventricle pumps oxygenated blood to the body.

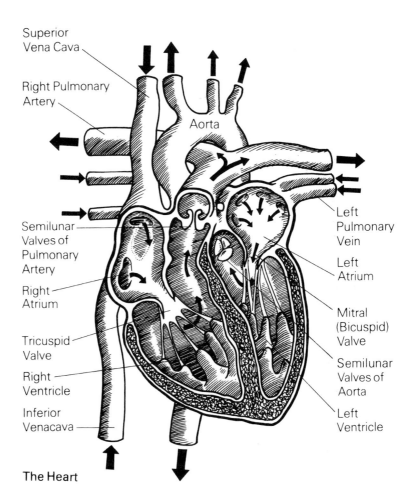

The Heart

The walls of the heart have three layers:

The Outer Pericardium is a strong protective membrane which holds the heart in position.
The Middle Myocardium is the muscular tissue.
The Inner Endocardium allows freedom of contraction and dilation by the middle layer.

In the Systemic System, deoxygenated blood enters the Right Atrium, passes through the tricuspid valve to the Right Ventricle and then through the Pulmonary Artery to the lungs. Gaseous exchange takes place in the alveoli. Blood returns through the Pulmonary Vein to the Left Atrium, through the mitral valve to the Left Ventricle and then out into the aorta to the body. In volume approximately 60 millilitres of blood are used each beat.

Volume of Blood Pumped by the Heart

The volume does not remain constant but varies with body activity. During vigorous exercise, the heart beats faster and its output increases. Much of the extra blood passes to the muscles and so provides them with the large amounts of oxygen that they need for their activity. The flow in each organ is controlled by the arterioles. When an organ is active the arterioles dilate allowing large amounts of blood to flow out of the arteries into the capillaries. When an organ is at rest the arterioles contract and the blood flow reduces.

Blood Pressure

Blood in the capillaries is under pressure, but this pressure is quite low, this can be seen when you cut yourself and bleed only a little. Blood in the artery is under much greater pressure and if an artery is cut the wound will bleed profusely. Blood pressure can be measured by using a sphygmomanometer and the level will rise during a contraction (Systole) and fall during relaxation (Diastole).

Average blood pressure, dependent upon age and fitness, is 120–80 Systole to 140–90 Diastole. It is usually recorded as a Systolic figure over the Diastolic e.g. $\frac{120}{80}$

Blood pressure serves two main purposes:
1 It impels some of the circulating blood upwards against gravity into the carotid arteries supplying blood to the brain.
2 It forces blood through the tiny capillaries in the tissues because these vessels are so narrow that the blood flow would be negligible without arterial pressure.

If it were not for blood pressure, the blood would gravitate to the lowest parts of the body.

The Heart and Circulation

The heart can be thought of as having two separate pumps. The two chambers on the right side of the heart supply blood at a low pressure to the lungs, via the pulmonary arteries. In the lungs the blood receives oxygen before returning it to the left side of the heart. The two chambers on the left side act as a high pressure pump, supplying blood via the arteries to the capillaries of the body. In the capillaries, oxygen passes from the blood to the tissues and carbon dioxide, a waste product of energy production, passes from the tissues into the blood. The blood is then collected in the veins and returned to the right side of the heart. Valves within the heart control the direction flow of the blood.

The heart is mainly muscle, which acts by contracting rhythmically. Each contraction causes a volume of blood to be pumped into the arteries. When the heart relaxes, blood flows into it from the veins. The amount of blood pumped out at each contraction will depend upon the volume of the lower chambers and the strength of the muscular contraction.

The Lungs and Circulation (Pulmonary System)

Average lungs will contain a total gas volume of approximately 5–6 litres, known as *total lung capacity*. However, at rest, only about 0.5 of a litre moves in and out of the lungs on each breath: this is the *tidal volume*. A normal breath out still leaves about 2.5 litres of air in the lungs. During exercise the tidal volume increases, both by having a bigger expiration and a bigger breath in (inspiration), until it may reach as much as 3 litres maximum. If you first give a maximum expiration and then measure the volume of a maximum inspiration, it will be about 4.5 litres. The volume obtained is called the *vital capacity*, which is the maximum volume of air that can be moved into or out of the lungs in one breath. The difference between the total lung capacity and the vital capacity is called the *residual volume* which represents the air which cannot be expelled from the lungs even by maximum expiration.

Effects of Exercise

During exercise the demand for oxygen increases. If the circulation (heart), and respiration (lungs), remain unchanged then there would be an increasing lack of oxygen for the working muscles. Lactic acid would continue to build up and the muscles would cease to function in a very short time.

The circulation and respiration rates are finely controlled to ensure that the supply of oxygen and food, together with the removal of carbon dioxide is maintained during exercise. These control processes are automatic and subconscious.

Aerobic and Anaerobic Energy Production

Energy is produced in the muscle in two ways.
1 Using oxygen or *aerobic energy*
2 Without oxygen or *anaerobic energy*

The level of activity relative to the fitness of the individual determines which of these two methods is used to produce the energy.

AEROBIC WORK

When the amount of oxygen taken up by the muscle is sufficient to supply the energy demanded by that muscle, energy is produced by the combustion of foodstuffs using oxygen, no harmful waste products result.

Aerobic respiration breaks down the carbohydrate or fat to give off energy, although the amount of oxygen required for this process differs. Fat requires more oxygen than carbohydrate and will give out more energy. Thus, when the oxygen supply is plentiful, fat will be burnt and when oxygen is less plentiful, as at the beginning and end of an aerobic workout, carbohydrate will be the fuel.

Aerobic activity, therefore, can be continued for a long time, for example, marathon running.

ANAEROBIC WORK

Energy for anaerobic work comes from two sources:
1 A ready made supply in the muscle (ATP and PC).
2 From the breakdown of carbohydrate without oxygen.

Anaerobic work demands energy immediately, for things like the final spurt at the end of a race, or squat thrusts in an exercise to music class.

The limiting factor in anaerobic work is the waste product produced. With aerobic work, harmless substances, water and carbon dioxide are left which are easily lost by the body. With anaerobic work, the carbohydrate is only partially broken down, and leaves a harmful substance called Lactic Acid, which builds up in the muscle causing fatigue. An individual working anaerobically, therefore, can only continue for a very short time.

Control of Circulation

The circulation rate is largely determined by the heart. The output from the heart or *cardiac output* is determined by multiplying the volume of blood ejected from the heart in each contraction, this is called *stroke volume*, by the number of strokes per minute or *heart/pulse rate*. When exercise occurs the heart rate increases from an average resting level of 60–70 beats per minute to as much as 180–200 beats per minute at maximum capacity. At the same time the heart will dilate slightly and contract more fully thus increasing the stroke volume. The cardiac output can in this way be increased by four or five times.

The supply of blood to areas of greatest demand during exercise can be further improved by selectively diverting blood away from non-active areas, such as the intestines and skin, and concentrating supplies to the active muscles.

If exercise is taken after a heavy meal the circulation finds itself in conflict as both the digestive system and the muscles demand blood to get oxygen. This causes a less than optimum result in both areas leading to a reduced exercise capability and possibly stomach cramps.

Control of Respiration

The level of respiration is found by multiplying the tidal volume and the rate of breathing (respiratory rate) and is measured in litres per minute.

At rest the breathing rate is normally 12–14 breaths per minute and the tidal volume about 0.5 litres. Therefore the level of expiration is 6–7 litres per minute. During exercise, the total expired rate and the tidal volume both increase so that the level of expiration may increase to 100–110 litres per minute.

At the end of an exercise period there is very rapid decreases in the rate of breathing, followed by a slower return to normal as the level of carbon dioxide in the body returns to normal.

THE RESPIRATORY SYSTEM

The Respiratory System consists of the organs used in breathing, for example, the Nose, Pharynx, Larynx, Trachea, Bronchii and Lungs. The job of the Respiratory System is to provide the blood with a constant supply of oxygen from the air and to allow unwanted carbon dioxide to be passed out of the blood back into the air. As you exercise, the efficiency of your Respiratory System is of critical importance. An inefficient system will render you relatively helpless or at least exhausted and unable to continue.

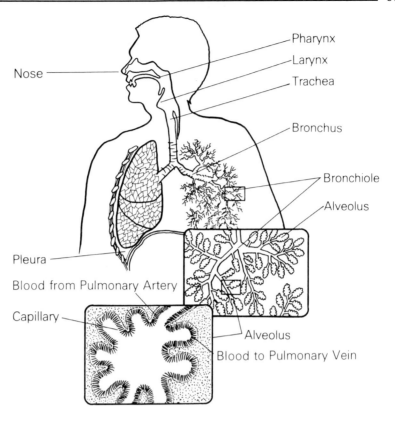

Organs of Respiration

The path by which air enters the lungs begins at the *nose* or the mouth. As a gateway through which air enters the body, the nose is more efficient than the mouth. It is divided by a vertical wall, the Septum, made of bone and cartilage. The cavities on each side are further divided into three narrow passages by bony ridges covered in a moist mucous membrane. This membrane moistens, warms and filters the air before it passes on to the lungs. The mouth is less efficient in moistening, warming and filtering the air.

The air then passes through the *pharynx*. This lies behind the nose and mouth and both cavities open into it. It receives both air and food. The lower end of the pharynx leads to the oesophagus in the front wall and enters the *larynx* or Adam's Apple. The cavity of the larynx is separated from the pharynx by a flap, the epiglottis, which prevents food from entering the windpipe. The lower part of the larynx leads into the *trachea* or windpipe, which is the main tube through which passes the air. It is cylindrical, ten or thirteen cm in length, and kept open by a series of rings of gristle or cartilage. These rings hold the trachea open enabling the air to flow freely. The *bronchii*, which next receive the air, are the two tubes into which the trachea divides at its lower end. One bronchus leads to each lung and then breaks up into smaller bronchii and even smaller bronchioles which serve every part of the lungs.

The *lungs* now receive the air. The two lungs are bulky organs which lie in the chest, one on each side of the heart. They have the appearance and texture of sponges. The right lung is divided into three lobes and the left into two. Each lobe is further divided into about 200 lobules and each lobule has many tiny air sacs or alveoli. Each alveolus has a corresponding bronchiole carrying air. Minute blood vessels carry carbon dioxide laden blood into the capillaries which surround each alveolus. The carbon dioxide passes through the single cell walls into the alveolus and is replaced by oxygen. This oxygenated blood is collected into veins and returned to the heart.

Breathing also involves the *diaphragm* which is a sheet-like muscle attached all round its edges to the lower part of the chest wall. It separates the chest from the abdomen. It is like an irregular dome which bulges into the chest. When it contracts it flattens, increasing the capacity of the chest cavity. At the same time the contents of the abdomen are pushed downwards causing the forward bulge. In addition, the short fibres of the *intercostal muscles* fill the space between the ribs. These slope so that when they contract the front part of the ribs and the sternum are moved upwards. As a result the diameter of the chest cavity is increased and thus its capacity is also increased.

The Effect of the Breathing Action

This is to expand the chest during inspiration or breathing in, causing the outer layer of the pleura of the lungs to be pulled outwards, reducing the pressure in the pleura space. To equalise the pressure, air passes into the lungs which expand and fill the extra space in the chest cavity. When the chest decreases in size, during expiration or breathing out, the pressure in the pleura space increases, and the air is driven out of the lungs to reduce it. This alternating action, contraction and relaxation, makes up the respiratory cycle which continues throughout life.

Breathing

Breathing or respiration goes on continuously and for much of the time unconsciously, and automatically controlled by the respiratory centre of the brain. The chief factor controlling the rate and depth of breathing is the concentration of carbon dioxide (CO_2) in the blood. The respiratory centre responds very quickly to slight changes in concentration of CO_2 and an increase of only 0.3 in the CO_2 content doubles the volume of air breathed in and out. Lack of oxygen also affects the breathing rate but is detected mainly by sensors in the large blood vessels in the neck. Each day an adult human breathes in and out approximately 25,000 times taking in about 600 cubic feet of air. From this about 22 cubic feet of oxygen passes into the alveoli and thence into the blood where it combines with the haemoglobin in the red corpuscles. It is thus carried to all parts of the body for use in providing energy.

Variations in Breathing

When sitting quietly, adults breathe approximately 14–20 times a minute to provide just sufficient oxygen for their bodies. (Babies breathe 30–40 times a minute: this slows as they grow up). The air taken in and out with each respiration is called *tidal air*. At rest this is usually 350–500 millilitres per breath of which about 150 millilitres only occupy the air passages and do not reach the lungs.

In *forced respiration*, a man breathing as deeply as possible can draw in about 3,500 millilitres, approximately 7 times more than normal. Alternatively if, at the end of a normal expiration, he tries to expel as much air as possible he can breathe out a further 1,000 millilitres by deliberate muscular effort.

If after breathing in as deeply as possible, a man breathes out as deeply as possible, the volume represents the greatest volume of air the lungs can exchange. It is called the *vital capacity* and varies between 3 and 5 litres in women and men. The 350 millilitres of air used at rest can be, with muscular effort, increased to 8,400 millilitres (i.e., ×24): similarly, the normal 14–20 breaths per minute may be increased to 80 per minute.

Pure, dry air contains 78% nitrogen, 21% oxygen, 1% argon and traces of other gases including 0.3% Carbon Dioxide. *Normal* air usually contains water vapour, dust, pollen, germs, poisonous gases and other pollutants and the carbon dioxide content is nearer 0.7%. The body's defence mechanisms work to prevent the unwanted substances reaching the lungs.

Malfunctions of the Respiratory System

Under normal conditions, the Respiratory System works so smoothly that we are not even aware of it. There are a number of illnesses which can affect the Respiratory System and make exercising uncomfortable and sometimes impossible.

1 The common cold obstructs breathing by causing watery mucous to collect in the nose and block the flow of the incoming air.
2 Bronchitis is an even more troublesome inflammation which obstructs the air flow by causing the lining of the airtubes to swell.
3 Asthma, often brought on by an allergy, anxiety or tension, can make muscles in the bronchi contract so that the victim continuously wheezes and gasps for air.
4 Tuberculosis can destroy the basic lung tissue thus preventing oxygen transportation.
5 Pneumonia inflames the lungs which fills the alveoli with a sticky substance that prevents the air from penetrating the membrane leading to the blood.
6 Emphysema involves the loss of elasticity in the alveoli resulting in over distension of the lungs.
7 Pneumoconiosis and asbestosis are occupational diseases caused by inhalation of toxic dusts.
8 Lung cancer may kill.

The Structure of a Class of Exercise to Music

Every class of exercise to music should have a structure that includes the following components:

1 Warm-Up
2 Aerobic
3 Muscular Strength & Endurance
4 Stretching
5 Cool-Down

The order in which these components are organised is open to some debate, and different interpretations, depending upon the attitude of the teacher, and the nature of the class.

We have found in our experience that the above order is generally most satisfactory to give class members an all-round workout. In addition, the duration of each component can be varied so that a class may be predominantly an Aerobic class, a Stretch class, a Strength and Endurance class or a general Keep Fit class. All of these components may be adjusted according to the fitness levels and ages of the participants.

WARM-UP

THE AIM OF A WARM-UP IS TO:

1 Prepare the joints for work.
2 Prepare the cardiovascular system for strenuous work by increasing the body temperature and blood flow to the working muscles.
3 Prepare the neuromuscular response patterns.
4 Prevent muscular soreness and injury.

THE WARM-UP SHOULD INCLUDE:

1 Exercises that flow from one to another and involve a graduation from those of a lesser to a greater intensity. (Mobility and loosening exercises is the best term to define these.)
2 Exercises that promote the circulation and include all body segments and major muscle groups.
3 Stretching exercises which are static in nature and held for approximately 8 seconds. These must follow activities described in points 1 and 2.
4 Activities that provide for a release of tension.
5 Exercises that are non-restrictive in nature, i.e. rhythmic, not jerky or bouncy exercises.

6 Exercises that gradually increase in intensity and avoid raising the heart rate rapidly.

7 Exercises that are suited to the individual and relate to the context of the class.

8 No time lag during the warm-up or before the next component.

9 Flexibility in the time allowed for the warm-up session from five to twenty minutes. The time allotted to the warm-up may decrease slightly with an increase in the fitness of students and in relation to the temperature conditions of the exercising environment.

YOU SHOULD APPRECIATE THAT:

1 The body temperature increases gradually.

2 There is an increase in the rate of exchange of oxygen from the blood to the tissues.

3 The body's blood vessels dilate due to an increase in the rate of blood flow. During exercise, in order to cope with the demand for extra oxygen, the body redistributes blood from relatively inactive tissues, and the digestion system, to voluntary muscles. Bearing this point in mind, it should be more understandable why it is not advisable to eat before an exercise session.

  The warm-up therefore gives the body time to transport the extra supply of blood to those areas that will need it during the later more strenuous sections of the exercise programme.

4 The body's heart, metabolic and respiratory rates are raised. If demands are made on the circulatory and respiratory systems gradually, you will feel little or no discomfort: therefore the warm-up assists physical efficiency.

5 As the supply of synovial fluid to the joints is increased and the deep muscle temperature is raised, the muscle fibres, ligaments, tendons and connective tissue become more pliable or flexible. Due to the structure of the joints all of these changes contribute to the increase in the range of movement of the joint, thereby protecting the body against injury.

6 There is an increase in deep muscle temperature which helps decrease viscosity (internal friction) within the muscles. Decreasing viscous resistance in the muscles allows the muscle to contract and relax with greater speed. By increasing the speed of muscle contraction and relaxation in the warm-up, the muscles are prepared for harder work without extra risk of injury.

7 Messages are sent from the brain to the rest of the body by a series of complex sensory and motor nerves. If the exercises during warm-up are related to the main part of the exercise session that is to follow, it will rehearse and facilitate selected neuromuscular response patterns. Although it is unreasonable to suggest that a warm-up improves skill it is fair to say that a warm-up may facilitate skillful movement.

8 You should be given the opportunity physiologically to prepare for the exercise session. You should be allowed to concentrate your thoughts on the task ahead and, as suggested in point 7

above, if the exercises are related you can mentally rehearse the routines. You will be less distracted and more absorbed in what the body is doing and therefore be more inclined to perform to the best of your ability.

APPROPRIATE EXERCISES FOR A WARM-UP SHOULD INCLUDE THE FOLLOWING MOVEMENTS:

a Flexion, extension and rotation of neck
b Flexion, extension, abduction, adduction of the shoulder girdle.
c Flexion, extension, rotation and circumduction of the shoulder joints.
d Flexion, extension and rotation of the trunk.
e Flexion, extension, abduction and circumduction of the hip joints (especially stretch the hamstring.
f Flexion, extension of the knees.
g Plantor flexion and dorsiflexion of the ankles (especially stretch the calves).

Remember:

1 The warm-up should include both stretching exercises and exercises that increase the activity of the heart and circulatory system.
2 To do lateral side bends in order to mobilise the back prior to forward flexion.
3 To keep the knees slightly bent (do not lock knees).
4 Not to do isometric exercises (resistive work, vigorous cardiovascular work and breath holding).

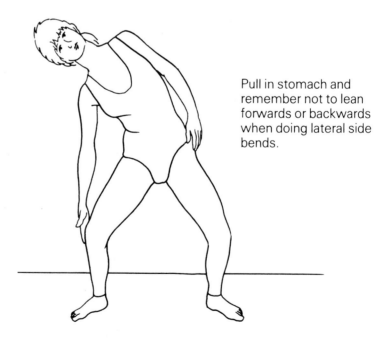

Pull in stomach and remember not to lean forwards or backwards when doing lateral side bends.

On the next page is a list of some mobilising exercises which may be done and the joints they involve:

NB: All exercises to be performed in a slow and controlled manner.

Joints involved	Mobility Exercises
Shoulders	Standing or sitting shoulder rolls. Standing or sitting hands on shoulders, circle elbows.
Elbows	Standing or sitting, hands to shoulders palms up, bend and straighten arms. Standing or sitting, hands to shoulders, rotate palms up and down.
Wrists	Standing or sitting, wrist circling. Standing or sitting, flex and extend wrist.
Neck	Standing or sitting, turn head to left and right. Standing or sitting, bend head forward and extend chin up (take care not to drop the head back).
Mid Spine	Hands and knees, hump and hollow. Hands and knees, circle trunk.
Waist	Standing side bending, hands on hips (knees slightly bent). Standing waist twists, hands on hips (take care to keep hips facing forward).
Lower Back	Standing pelvic circles (keep knees slightly bent) Lie on front, hands under shoulders, push shoulders and chest off floor (take care to keep hips on the floor).
Hips	Draw knee to chest, right and left alternate. Standing point toe forwards and backwards, and to the side.
Knees	Standing feet apart, bend knees.
Ankle	Standing or sitting ankle circling. Standing or sitting point and flex foot.

VARIETY AND PROGRESSION

It is quite difficult to create variety in a warm-up. The levels of preparation must remain fairly constant, even though the warm-up for an unfit middle-aged person will be different from that of a fit young athlete.

Different body starting positions can create variation and can be essential for the unfit, for example, lying or sitting on the floor or sitting in a chair.

AEROBIC
THE AIM OF AN AEROBIC SESSION IS TO:

1 Provide a controlled duration of exercise at the right level and for the right length of time in order to induce a cardiorespiratory training effect.
2 Improve the capacity and efficiency of the circulatory and respiratory system to deliver oxygen to the working muscles and to carry chemical waste products away at the same rate.

HOW IT IS DONE

1 Exercises should be provided that demand large amounts of oxygen to be transported to the tissues via the blood. Excellent examples of this are, running, swimming, cycling, jogging and dancing.

However, we are primarily concerned here with the area of exercise routines to music, so we will look for low tension activities which have a rhythmic nature and which use large muscle groups.

2 Activities are provided of a non-competitive nature, because a competitive situation may induce tension, create poor training habits or encourage too high a work load.

3 Proper work loads are assessed for each individual, by heart-rate monitoring, and close observation of the ability of the class to carry on a conversation during the aerobic session.

It is important for the exercise teacher to keep the intensity of the workout within your capacity. The most convenient way is to teach you how to take your pulse rate immediately after exercise, and use it as a guide. (See page 28.)

4 The aerobic training should be made progressive. In a beginners programme, the training progression is brought about by decreasing the resting interval between exercises while keeping the intensity constant. Beyond this level, both the resting interval and the intensity of exercise may be varied to produce the desired training effect.

5 Extra care should be taken with untrained middle-aged students. Very little exercise is needed to induce a training response with this group.

6 Jogging for beginners should begin at an approximate 10 minute mile pace. Walking, race walking, slow jogging and cycling are good for beginners as it is easy to control the exercise intensity so that people do not over-work themselves.

7 Directional changes should be included when you are jogging around a gym to prevent undue stress to one side of the body, caused by the mechanical effects of running a curved path.

8 Students should be encouraged to jog with a heel-toe, or flat foot strike and discouraged from landing on the ball of the foot or toes.

9 Suitable clothing should be worn. Rubberised or other impervious clothing should not be permitted. Correct footwear is of the utmost importance if leg soreness is to be avoided.

10 Vigorous aerobic activity should be gradually tapered-off before the next set of exercises. This will prevent blood pooling in the legs.

11 Endurance, not speed should be emphasised.

12 At least 20 minutes may be allotted to this component bearing in mind the beginners will need to build up to this level.

YOU SHOULD APPRECIATE THAT:

1 A low resting heart rate is not a good indicator of physical fitness.

There is a great variation in resting heart rates, the 'normal' ranging anywhere from 40 beats per minute to more than 90 beats per minute. The resting heart rate does decrease with training but this cannot be compared directly to the level of fitness because a low resting heart rate can be found in an untrained person, or a person who has a heart condition.

2 A variety of factors affect the heart rate during rest and exercise.

The heart rate can be affected by temperature, humidity, emotional tension, time of the day, time since previous meal, smoking and drugs.

If you use the heart-rate test, steps must be taken to dispense with as many of these variables as possible.

3 Recovery heart rate is related to exercise heart rate.

The heart rate begins to return towards resting values at the end of exercise. The speed at which it returns will depend primarily on the intensity of exercise, providing no other modifying effects are present. It is generally accepted that a quick recovery reflects a more efficient circulatory system.

If your teacher does not advise the taking of heart rates, it may be that she is unaware of the above facts. It is important for you to take and record your heart rate after the exercise session as well as before and during.

4 There is an increased blood flow during exercise.

During exercise the heart beats faster and the blood vessels dilate, allowing for the increased blood flow to the muscles. The working muscles produce a massaging or pumping action which accommodates this increased blood flow by speeding the return of blood to the heart.

If exercise is suddenly stopped this pumping action ceases, but the rate of blood flow into the muscles is still rapid. The result can be an accumulation or pooling of blood in the veins. The veins whose job it is to return used blood back to the lungs to be reoxygenated, have a valve system that prevents the backwards flow of blood, but during intense exercise the muscular pump action actually moves the blood back to the heart. Sometimes the amount of blood in the veins is so great that there is not enough blood returned to the heart for it to maintain an effective pumping pressure.

5 The demand for oxygen changes during exercise.

When the body begins exercise, there is immediately a greater demand by the muscles for oxygen. It takes a few minutes (2–5) for the cardiovascular system to adapt and consequently a feeling of discomfort often occurs. For example, the first few minutes of a run are always the hardest. Since there is insufficient oxygen at this time to provide energy aerobically, anaerobic respiration occurs and lactic acid is produced. Once the cardiovascular system has adapted to the new demands, aerobic respiration will predominate providing that the level of activity does not exceed an individual's aerobic capacity. An indicator of this level will be the ability to hold a conversation.

A thorough, but well graduated, warm-up will alleviate the initial discomfort when you exercise as the rate of increase of energy demand will be slow and therefore able to be met by aerobic respiration.

6 Through exercise the aerobic and anaerobic training system is being trained.

You can be said to be training your aerobic system when your heart rate is maintained above 60% of your maximum. As your heart rate increases, energy is provided in increasing amounts by the anaerobic system. When you are working at 85% you are reaching the capacity of your aerobic system and if your heart rate goes higher, you will be working almost totally anaerobically.

Anaerobic energy supply is more demanding and stressful on the body, although it will benefit your aerobic system.

Gentle jogging and skipping exercises will be aerobic exercise for the average individual. For the same individual, a routine that consists of gentle jogging, high leg kicks and squats will demand energy from the anaerobic system.

7 Lung function is related to performance.

As the intensity of aerobic exercise increases, the demand for oxygen and air increases. There is a very close relationship between the amount of oxygen used by the body and the pulmonary minute volume, which is the amount of air moved through the lungs per minute.

The maximum ventilation of the lungs improves with training, but it is not a limiting factor in exercise.

For example, untrained middle-aged men may be able to ventilate only 40–80 litres of air per minute. During hard exercise a normal male PE college student will ventilate about 120 litres per minute, while exceptionally good distance runners may be able to breathe over 200 litres per minute for brief periods of time.

APPROPRIATE AEROBIC EXERCISES SHOULD INCLUDE:

Running, swimming, cycling, jogging and dancing. As we are primarily concerned here with the area of exercise routines to music, your routines will incorporate running with rhythm, jogging, hopping and skipping and, depending upon personal taste, some dancing, in order to promote cardiovascular fitness.

VARIETY AND SAFE PROGRESSION ARE IMPORTANT ELEMENTS IN THE AEROBIC SESSION

Duration, frequency and intensity are three principles involved in all progressive exercise programmes.

When designing choreographed aerobic routines, care should be taken to frequently change the routines. Star jumps, high knee and leg kicks, strength exercises such as squat thrusts and burpees, should be included in progressively harder routines. Variety and progression can also be provided by increasing the number and repetitions of the exercises and by choosing faster music to which to work.

Your teacher ought to make you aware of forms of aerobic activity other than exercise to music. However well you are taught, there is a limit to the variety that can be given to you when the frequency with which you wish to exercise to music increases. You can often be revitalised in your exercise programme by becoming involved in a completely different form of aerobic activity, for example, jogging, swimming or cycling. Your perception of 'fitness' can be widened as you apply the exercise/fitness principles that you have learned to another area, and you can become further motivated.

MUSCULAR STRENGTH AND ENDURANCE

THE AIM OF A MUSCULAR STRENGTH AND ENDURANCE SESSION IS TO:

1 Make all the muscles strong enough to support the skeletal structure and to maintain posture and body shape.
2 Improve muscular endurance so that the body can take part in an activity that involves continuous use of the muscles whether it is for 45 minutes of gardening or 45 minutes of exercise to music.

THE MUSCULAR STRENGTH AND ENDURANCE SESSION SHOULD INCLUDE:

1 A progressive programme of strength exercises.
   A strength programme incorporates a low number of repetitions of an exercise with a comparatively high resistance.
2 A progressive programme of endurance exercises.
   An endurance programme incorporates a high number of repetitions of an exercise with a comparatively low resistance.
   NB: In both of the above programmes the exercises can be isotonic and isometric in nature. For a more detailed explanation, see Section C below.
3 Clear advice to follow in your progressive muscular strength and endurance programmes, for example:
   a Do not hold your breath while performing any exercises.
   b Exercises for all the major joint movements of the different body segments should be included.
   c You should not swing freely against a fixed joint, as this throws undesirable strain on muscles, tendons and ligaments, for example, forced toe touching by bouncing when your knees are locked.
   d You should maintain a high level of activity without creating local fatigue by shifting forceful work from muscle group to muscle group. For example, more than two consecutive sets of stomach exercises in a beginners class is inadvisable. The exercises should be arranged so that the muscles are allowed to relax and rest between sets.
   e There should be minimal hesitation when moving from one exercise to another.
   f Encouragement to work at your own level.
4 Exercising for 10–15 minutes duration.

WHEN PERFORMING MUSCULAR STRENGTH AND ENDURANCE EXERCISES YOU SHOULD APPRECIATE THAT:

1 *Isotonic Exercise* is dynamic moving exercise, performed while breathing freely, which builds strength throughout the full range of movement. It incorporates two types of muscle contraction, concentric, which produces a shortening of the muscle, and eccentric which produces a lengthening of the muscle.
2 *Isometric Exercise* involves no movement of body parts or muscle length changes and is also known as 'static contraction'.

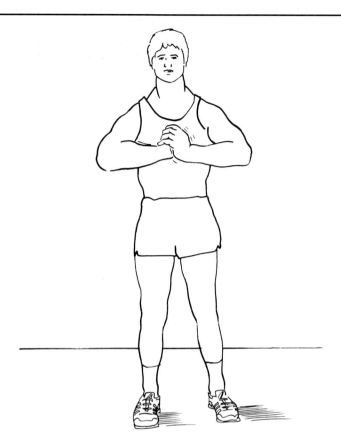

Isometric contraction of the chest by pressing the palms together.

Isotonic Training gives:

1 More muscle growth and better capilliarization increases than isometric training.
2 Strength more evenly throughout the full range of movement.
3 Better nerve-muscle co-ordination as a result of more complex actions.
4 A strength increase more readily applied to actual exercise performance.

Isometric Training:

1 Requires less time, less energy, less space and in some cases little or no equipment.
2 Can improve muscular strength quickly but it has a number of limitations.
  a It increases strength only in the position performed and not throughout the full range of movement.
  b It can produce muscle strain if prolonged.
  c It produces a high increase in blood pressure relative to heart rate and thus a possible reduction in the oxygen supply to the heart and brain.
Consequently, isometric exercises should not be used when working with unfit adults. It is better to use isotonic exercises

because they have all the necessary qualities to produce muscular strength and endurance without the above limitations.

Correct breathing in relation to exercise is important because:

During a strength programme, particularly one concerned with Weight Training, or Weight Lifting an emphasis on correct breathing techniques will help to avoid the onset of something called the Valsalva Effect. This can occur when you strain to lift a weight or move an object whilst holding your breath. Such action will create pressure in the chest cavity and an increase in blood pressure which can lead to decreased blood flow to the brain causing fainting. This effect can be avoided by breathing out during the *straining* part of the exercise.

APPROPRIATE EXERCISES FOR MUSCULAR STRENGTH AND ENDURANCE INCLUDE:

1 Toe tapping for the front of the lower leg.
2 Jogging for the calves.
3 Lateral leg raise for the lateral thigh.
4 Half squat for the thighs and buttocks.

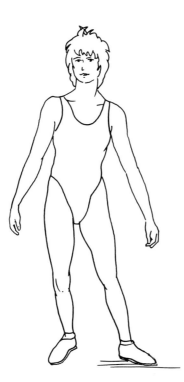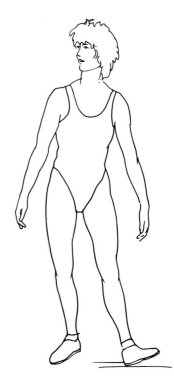

Toe tapping
Lift the toe as high as possible.

5 Press-ups for the posterior arms, anterior chest. (You should remember to do easy press-ups, against a wall if a beginner.)
6 Bent knee sit-ups, bending the trunk forward, for the abdominals.
7 Crunches, (sit-ups) curling the shoulders off the floor with a twist for the abdominals.
8 Single leg raises, lying on your front, for the buttocks and back of the thigh.

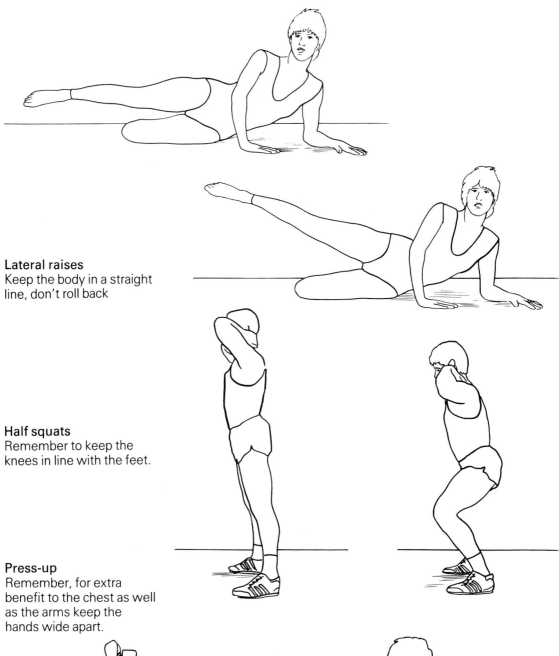

Lateral raises
Keep the body in a straight
line, don't roll back

Half squats
Remember to keep the
knees in line with the feet.

Press-up
Remember, for extra
benefit to the chest as well
as the arms keep the
hands wide apart.

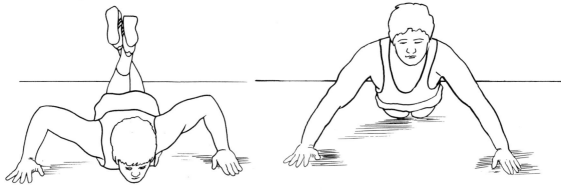

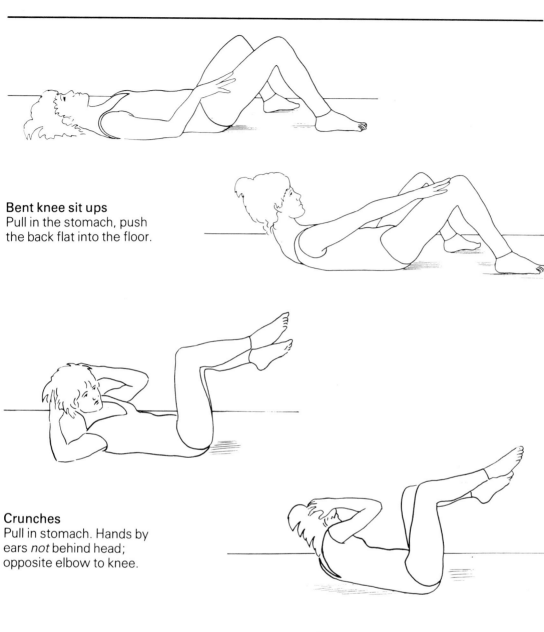

Bent knee sit ups
Pull in the stomach, push
the back flat into the floor.

Crunches
Pull in stomach. Hands by
ears *not* behind head;
opposite elbow to knee.

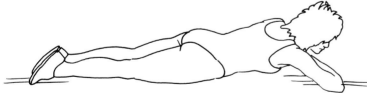

Single leg raises
Keep chin and hips on
floor and raise leg slowly.

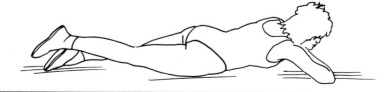

THE MAJOR MUSCLES AND MUSCLE GROUPS (See diagrams pages 42/43)

MUSCLE	POSITION	ACTION	EXERCISE
TRAPEZIUS	Triangular shaped muscle across the back of neck and shoulders.	Draws shoulders together and downwards, generally acts as brace for shoulders. Bad tone in the Trapezius can lead to round shoulders. (The Trapezius takes a lot of strain if you sit hunched over a desk or a typewriter for long hours.)	Shoulder circling and controlled arm movements. Arms front horizontal position to overhead position or shoulder shrugs.
DELTOIDS	Over the top of the shoulder joints like epaulettes.	Raise arms sideways and in conjunction with other muscles help rotate the arms and raise them to the front and back.	Any arm raising movement or lifting weights. Lifting the humerus from side position to horizontal e.g. star jumps. Sports like gymnastics, climbing, tennis are also good.
LATISSIMUS DORSI	The broad muscle which stretches across the back into the back of the arms.	Helps draw arms down and back and to rotate them. Also pulls trunk up towards static arms (as in rope climbing).	Any pulling movement against resistance. Sports like rowing and climbing are good.
PECTORALS	Upper chest.	Help draw the arms across the body and rotate arm inwards. In women they support the breasts.	Press-ups with hands wide, throwing and serving in tennis. Strong resistance of the hands against an immovable object. Clasping hands in front of your chest and pushing inwards.
BICEPS	Front of the upper arm.	Bends the arm. Turns palm upwards when arm is bent.	Arm-bending movements, against a resistance, e.g. pull-ups and arm curls with weights.
TRICEPS	Back of the upper arm.	Straighten the elbows.	Pushing arms against resistance, push-ups are an excellent exercise.
ILIOPSOAS	Two muscles connecting part of the lower spine and hip bone to the top of the thigh.	Flexes the hip. Turns the thigh outwards. When the thigh is fixed the iliopsoas muscle pulls on the spine and at the thigh to flex the hip as in rising to a sitting position from the supine position.	Raising and lowering a single leg while lying on the back (the other leg should remain bent and foot flat to the floor). Running activities, with the legs lifted high.

MUSCLE	POSITION	ACTION	EXERCISE
HAMSTRINGS (Semitendinosus) (Semimembranosus) (Biceps Femoris)	Back of thigh.	Bend the knees and help to turn them outwards and extend the legs backwards. The hamstrings are particularly vulnerable; as exercise such as walking and sitting do not exercise them enough.	Leg flexing and extending a straight leg backwards.
ABDOMINALS (Rectus Abdominis, Internal, External Obliques, Transversus Abdominis)	A muscular 'corset' three layers thick joining the bottom of the ribs to the top of the pelvic girdle.	Bend the trunk forwards and from side to side. Rotate the trunk and support the stomach. Strong abdominals give a flat, firm stomach.	By curling up against a resistance. By performing sit-ups and/ or touching opposite elbow to knee.
QUADRICEPS (Rectus Femoris, Vastus Medialis, Vastus Lateralis, Vastus Intermedius).	Front of thigh	Extend the knees and bend the hips.	Leg straightening and kicking movements. Cycling, climbing, running and walking are all good.
GLUTEALS Gluteus Maximus Gluteus Medius Gluteus Minimus (Buttocks)	A group of muscles which extend all over the seat.	Pull thighs sideways and backwards. They also rotate the legs and some of the muscles in the group help raise the trunk from a stooping position.	By raising leg backwards and by static contraction. By running, hopping, skipping and squatting.
GASTROCNEMIUS, SOLEUS (Tibialis Anterior, Tibialis Posterior) (Calves)	Back of lower legs.	Raise heels and point toes downwards.	Heel raising and toe pointing, standing on tip-toes, walking, running, jumping, dancing and hopping.
ADDUCTORS (Adductor Magnus, Adductor Longus, Adductor Brevis and Gracilis)	Inside of the thighs.	Pull legs inwards.	From lying on the side parallel with the floor, lift the lower leg against the line of gravity. Other exercises are pushing legs tightly together, riding and swimming (breast stroke).
ABDUCTORS (Tensor fascial latae, Gluteus Medius, Gluteus Minimus Sartorius)	Outside of the thighs.	Carry leg outwards and rotate it inwards.	Lateral raising of the leg.
TIBIALIS ANTERIOR	Front of the lower leg.	Pulls the foot upwards.	Toe tapping, ankle circling and eversion of the foot.

PROGRESS IN ORDER TO FURTHER IMPROVE MUSCULAR STRENGTH AND ENDURANCE CAN BE ACHIEVED THROUGH:

The use of weights. However, this method is not always practical in the class situation. It can be made feasible if the class make their own weights, or buy the fashionable light weights, such as 'heavy hands' or 'strap on' weights. Your teacher can also give you a weight training schedule to do in your own time, or encourage you to attend a special weight training course. The exercise class and weight training class would compliment each other, provide variation, and motivation for you to exercise more than once or twice a week.

You can make weights by filling some stocking material with beans, lentils, split peas etc. The weight used should depend on your sex, age, health and state of fitness.

Pages 68–69 contain a number of examples of muscle groups, their position, the action they perform, and the appropriate related exercise. You can use all of these provided they are performed correctly and that the body is prepared.

STRETCHING

THE STRETCHING COMPONENT SHOULD AIM TO:

1 Reduce muscle tension and make the body feel more relaxed.
2 Increase the range of movement of joints and muscles so that the body can work faster and more efficiently.
3 Prevent muscle soreness or muscle tears.
4 Eliminate muscle inflammation and facilitate recovery from soft tissue injuries.
5 Improve exercise technique by extending the rage of body movement.
6 Lengthen the muscle again after use.

NB: You help return the body to a non-exercising state when incorporating stretching exercises within the cool-down component.

HOW IT IS DONE

1 Your teacher should start the stretching routine by promoting a feeling of relaxation.
2 You should begin to stretch only after the muscles are warmed-up.
3 You should ease into the stretch to the point where it is comfortable and not painful. This is referred to as slow, static stretching.
4 You should stretch so that the pull is felt in the bulky, central, portion of the muscle. You should be asked to concentrate on relaxing the muscle or muscle groups being stretched.
5 You should not bounce in to the end of the range of movement of the joint.
6 You should not hold your breath, but try to breathe calmly and rhythmically.

7 You should try to stretch whenever possible in either sitting or reclining positions.

8 The choice of stretching exercises should be related to the aerobic and muscular strength and endurance component.

9 You need to stretch daily if gains in flexibility are to be achieved.

10 You should not compete during stretching exercises. You should not compare your progress with that of someone else. Trying too hard can lead to injury and result in the loss of any gains made. A feeling of mild discomfort during stretching is all that is needed.

11 You should alternate the stretching exercises from one muscle group to another, ensuring that they are progressive.

12 If you are an exceptionally flexible person, you should take a great deal of care not to stretch too far because there is a danger of injury through dislocation.

SHORT STRETCH COMPONENT

All major muscle groups should be stretched for 8-10 secs in order to prepare the muscles for work and prevent possible injuries.

DEVELOPMENTAL STRETCH COMPONENT

To promote an increase in flexibility, stretches need to be developed. You should hold the stretch for between 10-30 secs. As the feeling of tension within the muscle eases, you should develop the stretch further, ensuring you are stable, relaxed and comfortable.

WHEN PERFORMING STRETCHING EXERCISES YOU SHOULD APPRECIATE THAT:

Lack of flexibility and inefficient technique are the most frequent causes of poor physical performance as well as a reason for many strains and tear injuries in sport. Even today, the flexibility section of most training programmes is neglected. Athletes and keep-fit performers prefer to do strength and endurance work because in their minds they feel these components are doing them more good. What should be aimed for is a balanced programme, incorporating all five aspects of physical fitness.

It is believed that the myotatic reflexes play an important part in developing greater flexibility. Myotatic reflexes are the stretch reflex and the inverse stretch reflex.

STRETCH REFLEX

Whenever a muscle is stretched, the stretch reflex action automatically contracts the stretched muscle, in order to protect it from being overstretched. The stretch reflex action occurs in both a slow stretch and a jerky stretch. If a muscle is stretched quickly, the resulting contraction is likely to be more forceful than if the muscle is stretched gently and slowly. A quick, forceful stretch is more likely to lead to injury.

INVERSE STRETCH REFLEX

The inverse stretch reflex occurs within contracted and stretched muscles. When a muscle contracts or stretches, considerable tension develops in the muscle. The inverse reflex relaxes the muscle, in an attempt to prevent over-stretching of the muscle tissue. Therefore, if a stretched position is sustained at a high tension for long enough a point is reached where the tension dissipates and the muscle can be stretched even further. This phenomenon is due to the golgi tendon organ, or in layman's terms inverse stretch reflex.

Stretching may be performed ballistically or statically.

BALLISTIC

The ballistic stretching technique is performed with jerky or bouncing movement when the force of jerking and bouncing stretches the muscles. This technique invokes a strong stretch reflex contraction, thereby creating a great deal of muscle tension. Stretching a muscle against this amount of tension increases the chance of injury to the muscles and tendons and joints. The position is never held, so that muscles never get a chance to relax.

STATIC

In static stretching, the stretch position is assumed slowly and gently, and held ideally for 30 to 60 seconds. By doing this, the contraction from the stretch reflex is slow and mild. As the position is held the tension from the stretch eases allowing the muscles being stretched to be taken a little further, thus allowing an increase in flexibility.

Static stretching may be performed actively or passively.

Active

Active static stretching depends on strength in certain muscle groups, in order to adopt the necessary stretch position, e.g. a shoulder stretch with arms raised straight above the head. To achieve a stretch in the shoulder joint arms have to be extended up and back, hence muscles at the back of the shoulder and at the top of the back have to contract and work hard against the stiffness of the joint and resistance of the stretching muscles at the front. These stretched muscles need to relax. The ability to isolate particular muscle groups in order to contract the working muscles and to relax the stretching muscles, is necessary for this technique to work; a difficult skill. Consequently active stretching in this way is a limited method of producing great gains in flexibility. It is good however for building up strength in muscles surrounding a joint which is already particularly flexible. This will thus add to the stability of that joint in its extreme ranges of movement.

Passive

Passive stretching technique uses external force such as that of gravity or a partner to increase flexibility. All muscles of the limb and surrounding the joint involved in the stretch are thus able to relax totally. When done improperly or carelessly, it is easy to stretch the muscles and tendons beyond their limits and thus cause injury.

(Compared with other techniques passive stretching produces the least amount of tension and so is the most effective method of improving flexibility).

Stretching exercises should take into account the following parts of the body:

1 Shoulders
2 Neck
3 Arms
4 Chest
5 Abdominals
6 Back
7 Gluteals (buttocks) and hips
8 Groin and inner thighs
9 Hamstrings
10 Quadriceps
11 Calf
12 Ankles

However, always remember to select the stretching exercises that are best related to the activity which is to follow and always choose to do the easy stretching exercises first.

VARIETY AND PROGRESSION SHOULD BE CREATED IN A STRETCH SESSION

When stretching is first introduced it has to be taught with great care. Many people, particularly men, are naturally inflexible and therefore stretching does not come easily to them and if done incorrectly can be harmful.

Your beginners' exercise to music classes should include, in both warm-up and cool-down, simple stretching exercises which stretch out the essential muscles of the body, for example, the shoulder, waist, groin, hamstring, calf and quads. As you progress in your class, you can hold the stretches longer, even for up to 30 seconds. It is possible eventually to have the major part of your class made up of stretching routines. The key points for progression are:

1 Hold the stretches for longer.
2 Incorporate more exercises.
3 Incorporate more difficult exercises.
4 Do your own flexibility exercises every day.

Some of you may find stretch routines rather slow and boring, particularly when stretch positions are being held for 30 seconds. Your teacher's choice of music, approach to teaching and creativity in making up a sequence, will be vital in creating variety in the flexibility component.

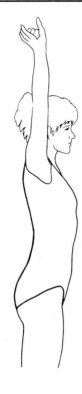

The diagrams (labelled 1, 2 below) show a progression in difficulty of stretch exercises.

Remember these are only suggestions. Stretching is very individual, only perform exercises that are comfortable for you. These positions should be held not bounced.

Shoulder stretch
1 Pull the stomach in.

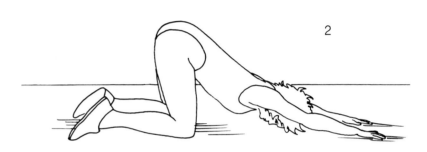

2

Groin stretch
1 Hold round the ankles.

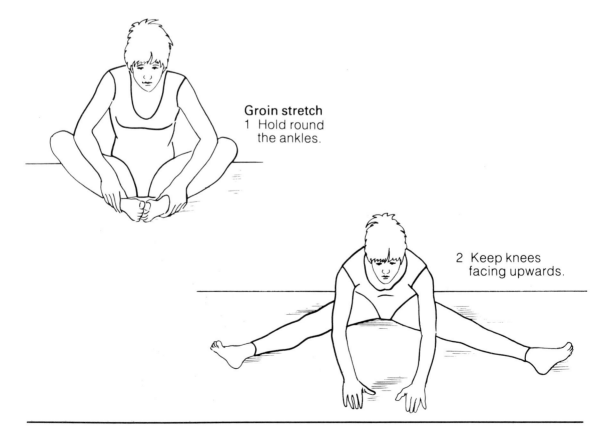

2 Keep knees facing upwards.

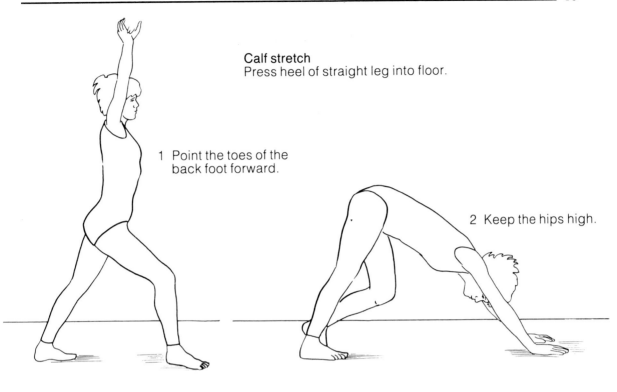

Calf stretch
Press heel of straight leg into floor.

1 Point the toes of the
back foot forward.

2 Keep the hips high.

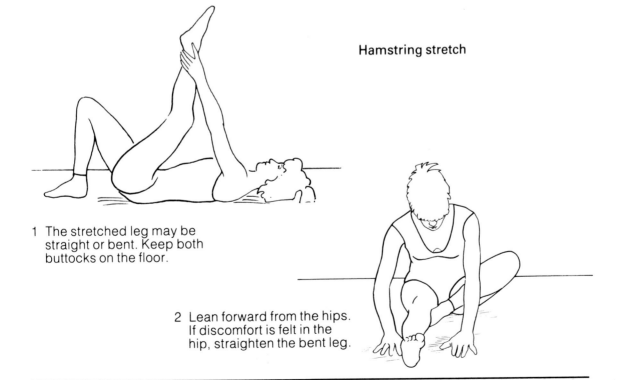

Hamstring stretch

1 The stretched leg may be
straight or bent. Keep both
buttocks on the floor.

2 Lean forward from the hips.
If discomfort is felt in the
hip, straighten the bent leg.

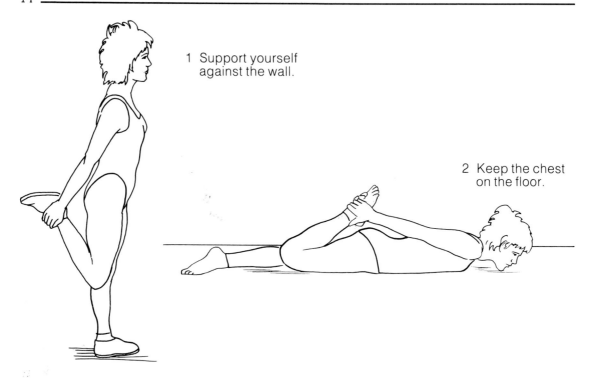

1 Support yourself against the wall.

2 Keep the chest on the floor.

COOL-DOWN AND RELAXATION

A COOL-DOWN AND RELAXATION SESSION SHOULD AIM TO:

1 Return the body gradually to the non-exercising state.
2 Relax in order to reduce physical tension.
3 Assist the circulatory system of the body to remove substances that may contribute to muscle stiffness or soreness.
4 Assist the circulatory system to help control adequate venous return and adequate cardiac output – thereby preventing possible dizziness or fainting after intense exercise.
5 Relate to the latest component of the class performed. Cool-down is not only appropriate for the end of the class but for each section.

COOL-DOWN AND RELAXATION CAN BE ACHIEVED BY:

1 Performing a mild rhythmic-activity.
2 Emphasising relaxing exercises to be performed in a non-stressful fashion.
3 Performing exercises which promote the return of blood from the extremities to the heart.
4 Allowing sufficient time to ensure that the heart rate recovers adequately by the end of the cool-down period relative to the fitness level of the individual.
5 Spending 5–10 minutes on this part of the class.

TO UNDERSTAND HOW THE BODY REACTS IN A COOL-DOWN YOU SHOULD APPRECIATE THAT:

1 When the activity period is over, many adaptions must be made during the process of recovery before the body returns to normal. This return is not instantaneous, but gradual. In the warm-up section it was explained why the body needs a period of time

to prepare for strenuous exercise. It is equally important that time is taken to cool-down after exertion.

2 After the exercise session, showers or baths should be warm rather than hot. The vasodilation (vein dilation), associated with exercise may be increased after a hot bath or shower, and this may lead to hypotension (low blood pressure), possible irregular heart beats, and even dizziness and fainting. This should not be a problem with most people but if it is, the water should be at a moderate temperature and time spent in it should be short.

3 Sauna and steam baths are not advisable immediately after an exercise work-out. The body will be exposed to increased heat at a time when it is trying to reduce its temperature. The body during exercise, loses fluid and this water loss continues during a sauna or steam bath and can reach danger levels of dehydration.

APPROPRIATE EXERCISES FOR COOL-DOWN AND RELAXATION SHOULD INCLUDE:

1 Mild jogging, skipping and walking to help promote venous return after the body has been involved in strenuous exercise.

2 A variety of stretching exercises to lengthen the muscles again which have shortened due to strenuous work.

3 Easy rhythmic flowing exercises such as arm swings, arm reaches forward, arm reaches to the side, knee bends and low knee lifts, are appropriate. Any mobility or loosening exercises that help to reduce the muscle and joint tension that is created during strenuous exercise are also recommended.

4 All types of relaxation exercises. During a period of relaxation the body learns to recognise tension and dispel it both locally and generally. You should isolate particular muscles and groups of muscles, and aim to relax them, by alternate tensing and relaxing exercises.

With careful planning and choreography the cool-down can have variety and interest.

Your preparation for the warm-up and the cool-down should take your entire body into account.

When considering progression or variation of a cool-down, your level of fitness, the environmental conditions, the time of day and the severity of your class must be taken into account.

7 The Use of Music

Selecting music for exercise is both difficult and time consuming; it is necessary to listen to as much variety as possible from records, tapes, concerts and radio, and to try and relate exercises in terms of musical rhythm and tempo. If a teacher has a pianist, some of the responsibility can be delegated provided that there is a great deal of co-operation between pianist and teacher.

CHOICE OF MUSIC

A teacher should decide on an exercise – its speed and duration in relation to the level of the class – and then select the appropriate music. If the selection is done in this order, there will be less possibility of the music dictating the programme of exercise rather than vice-versa. The beat of music is critical. Both teachers and students should listen to the music and mentally count regular beats. Sometimes this is not an easy exercise and is helped by tapping with a finger or clapping hands whilst counting to determine the natural and regular beat, for example, 1.2.3 1.2.3, 1.2.3.4 1.2.3.4 or 1.2 1.2.

The choice of music should reflect the ability and the level of fitness of the class. If you cannot follow the tempo of the music chosen by your teacher, a poor choice has been made.

You should have variety in your class, a variation in tempo can help in this respect, because certain components of the class may be suited to fast or slow tempo. In addition, a change of tempo can be as motivating for you as a change in music.

Different rhythms also create variety, for example, 1.2.3, 2.2.3 3.2.3 4.2.3, 1234 2234 3234 4234

Waltz or 3/4 time is suitable for dance and mobility exercises while 4/4 time is suitable for most types of exercise. 4/4 time is used in a lot of popular music and is a rhythm with which it is relatively easy to work.

The type of music used is virtually inexhaustible. However, when vocal music is used it is better that the voice on the tape or record is not too prominent otherwise it will compete with and perhaps dominate the teacher.

Orchestral or single instrument music has to be used carefully, as does big band music, because the beat often changes within one piece and so it is difficult to choreograph. On the whole, however, there should be no reason why you should become bored with the music as there is a wide choice available. It is also acceptable, at times, for your teacher to turn off the music and rely upon the voice to motivate and give rhythm to sustain the class.

The Selection of Music
THE WARM-UP

The selection of music for the warm-up can be particularly important because if you start with the right mental attitude to exercise it will motivate you to work well for the rest of the class.

A variety of rhythms and tempos can be used for this section, though when first mobilising the joints you should perform the exercises with control. However, if lively music is selected the teacher should count at half the dictated speed, so that, for example, in performing shoulder rolls, the exercise will not be too jerky. As your body gets warmer and the mobilising exercises become more flowing and rhythmic in nature, the teacher can use slightly faster beats incorporating walking, marching, easy skipping and jogging exercises. Having ensured that the body is completely warm, stretching exercises can be included. It may be necessary to choose music that has a slower beat because very lively music at this stage may encourage bouncing into stretched positions or ballistic stretching. Remember that it is advisable to perform static stretching at all times.

THE AEROBIC SECTION

This section is often the part that you enjoy the most. Even if the beginner has difficulty jogging or running, the music still needs to be vigorous, beaty and lively. The body is working hard at this stage, large amounts of oxygen are being pumped around the body, and therefore it is important that your teacher has selected music that will create a fun atmosphere to motivate you to keep working.

As you become fitter, you will be able to cope with a greater variety of speeds and rhythms. For example running, skipping and galloping are quite acceptable exercises. Teachers who are more familiar with dance step rhythms may incorporate different types of steps or even dance routines to provide variety. It is wise to remember that the teacher has to be sure that the exercises and the music are within the capabilities of your group because the class members can easily be carried along with the atmosphere, and end up utterly exhausted, and vow never go to an exercise to music class again!

MUSCULAR STRENGTH AND ENDURANCE

During this section, particularly when dealing with strengthening exercises, the music should be much slower than in the aerobics section, but not as slow as in the stretching section. The music should have a steady beat and perhaps a mellow vocal will add to the feeling of continuity and consistency. The fitter the group, the more lively the music may become, particularly when working on improving muscular endurance. However, the speed of the music should always match the exercise and the class should be able to cope with it. It is worth remembering that an exercise can be done at different speeds to the same piece of music by counting two or three beats together to slow down or half beats to speed up.

STRETCHING AND COOL-DOWN

During the final phase of the exercise class, music can help to return the body to a non-exercise state. The cool-down needs to use less vigorous music, but have a rhythmic nature to complement easy mobilising type exercises. However, when the cool-down includes stretching and relaxation exercises, the body moves into slow, controlled and held positions and the music can be slower.

Although you may tend to feel that because you are moving slowly, these type of exercises are not beneficial, you should appreciate that flexibility and relaxation exercises are an important and integral part of the exercise to music class.

THE IMPORTANCE OF MUSIC

The use of music is important for a variety of reasons. However, you should never allow the quality of your movement to suffer because you are engrossed in the music itself. To some extent your teacher can help in this respect by walking around the class and correcting individuals.

It is often better not to do an exercise at all than to do it incorrectly. Music is an aid, it should not be a distraction, and both you and your teacher should ensure that this is the case.

To give you a clear insight into how a teacher can phrase a piece of music, and link it with movement, we will try and show you, with this specific example of a well-known and easily available piece of music. In order to follow these steps, you will need to listen to this piece of music itself.

Record – *Help* The Beatles
1 Listen to the piece of music several times to establish a regular beat.
2 Count the music into 8 counts and record on paper, for example:
88888888888888888888888888

(It is important to realise that not all pieces of music will divide up into regular 8's, there may be occasional 4 or 2 counts.)
3 Once you are certain you have accurately broken down the music, in this case 27 sets of 8, listen and try to group together those 8 counts that make up a phrase of the music.
88 88 88 88 88 88 88 88 88 88 88 88 88 8

(Try to think of a phrase as a sentence. It is important to realise that not all musical phrases consist of pairs of 8's.)
4 Repeat the above but indicate which phrases sound the same.

Intro	A	A	B	B1	A	A	B	B1	C	D	B	B1	E
88	88	88	88	88	88	88	88	88	88	88	88	88	8

A B C D E represent the different phrases of the music. (B1 means the phrase is basically B with a slight difference.)

5 Having identified the pattern of phrases within the music, e.g. Intro (introduction) AA BB1 AA BB1 CD BB1 E, select appropriate exercises to fit the character of each phrase of music.

Intro   Jogging on the spot.

A   8 twisting backwards and 8 jogging forward.

B   skipping on spot, 4 alternate arms high and 4 alternate arms low (8 counts) and repeat

B1   skips as B (8 counts) then 2 double arm circles bending knees (8 counts)

C   Lunge to the Right and to the Left, with your arms above your head (4 counts) and repeat

D   twists 8 to the Right, 8 to the Left (8 counts)

E   Double arm circle bend knees (2 counts) 4 times in all.

6 The routine will then fit together as follows.

Phrase	Number of beats	Exercise
Intro	16	jogging on the spot
A	16	twists and jogs
A	16	twists and jogs
B	16	skipping
B1	16	skipping and arm circles
A	16	twists and jogs
A	16	twists and jogs
B	16	skipping
B1	16	skipping and arm circles
C	16	lunges (4)
D	16	twists 8 to right and 8 to left
B	16	skipping
B1	16	skipping and arm circles
E	8	arm circles

7 Having followed these stages, you will have created a choreographed movement sequence. Many teachers do not go into this amount of detail and it is quite acceptable to follow the general beat of the music. The teacher selects 3 or 4 exercises that match the music and then repeats them throughout the piece of music regardless of any chorus or vocal or instrumental changes. This use of music is obviously not as time consuming and allows an experienced teacher the opportunity to ad-lib in the choice of exercise. However, the more choreographed method can become quite easy for the experienced teacher and more enjoyable for the teacher and the class. Once the class goes beyond the beginners stage, they too will relate exercise to music. Choreographed routines also promote class confidence and enjoyment.

Exercise to Music and its Contribution to Physical Fitness

Whether you have already started or are thinking of starting to take part in exercise, you should be aware of some general guidelines related to all exercise programmes.

Are you ready to take part in exercise?

1 Are you generally in good health and seldom ill, if not you should consult your doctor before you start exercising. Have you any idea how unfit you are? If you have no idea, then perhaps, after reading chapters 3 and 4, you could take a physical fitness assessment test.

2 Your exercise programme should be designed to increase your level of physical fitness slowly, where other people jog, you might have to walk; where other people continue for 20 minutes in an aerobic session, you may perhaps do only 10 minutes.

3 Whatever your starting point, your fitness programme should be progressive with a steady increase in the workload and no dramatic increases under any circumstances.

4 Before taking part in an exercise to music class, find out at what level of fitness it is directed. The advertisement or publicity should give you some indication. For example, if it may say 'Fitness Classes to Music, aimed at those under 40 at present involved in some kind of physical activity once a week', or 'aimed at those over 60 who have not exercised for some time'. This information is a fair indication that the teacher is aware of different levels of fitness.

General factors relating to different fitness levels

1 COMPETITION AND RECREATION

There is a difference between playing a sport competitively, particularly at higher levels, and playing a sport recreationally. Competitive football, rugby, squash and swimming, etc require some degree of physical fitness and also produce fitness when performed. Recreational games and sports, however, usually do not *develop* fitness. If you are physically fit then it is more likely that you will be able to both enjoy your recreational sport more, and also perform more safely.

Recreational activities are obviously better than doing nothing. Walking for the old and unfit person could improve cardiovascular fitness. However, a fit 40-year-old would have to walk quickly to increase her heart rate to produce an effective training gain and some people may prefer an even more beneficial fitness class.

2 PRINCIPLES OF TRAINING

You should consider several principles of training when planning your exercise programme.

a Duration, Frequency and Intensity

Duration, frequency and intensity are the three principles involved in all progressive exercise programming. How often, how long, and how hard should you exercise? A summary of many studies indicates that physiological changes will occur and you will obtain significant benefit if you exercise three times a week. This is not to say that exercising less frequently than this will not be good for you, rather that the physiological benefits will be less.

Of course, there are some of you who will wish to exercise more than three times a week. You will have to ensure that joints and muscles are not overworked and that injury is not sustained. It is possible to become obsessive about your exercise which is not really a healthy state of mind, particularly if you are thereby put off exercise by the pressure that you put upon yourself. Under these circumstances, a variety of different kinds of exercise would be recommended, so that you do not become bored.

b Overload

To promote physiological improvement and bring about a training effect, a specific exercise overload must be applied. This is achieved by exercising at a level above normal, which may be reached by increasing the frequency, intensity, or duration of exercise.

PLATEAUING

The 'plateauing' effect that occurs when fitness improves or a skill is acquired, and can happen after a few weeks or a few months. When you reach this levelling-off standard and you start to think that you will no longer improve, it is the teacher's job to assure you that this is normal and that if you continue exercising, practising the skill, or vary the type of activity, progress will be made.

d Specificity

Training is specific. Each sport develops its own particular kind of fitness. Exercise to music, however, should give you a general overall fitness.

e Individual Differences

Few people show the same response to training. Several factors are responsible, including:

i Different fitness levels at the start of training.
ii Physiological differences including body type and muscle type.
iii Varying levels of skill.
iv Motivation of the individual.

It is unrealistic to expect all participants to respond to a given training dosage in precisely the same way. Training benefits are best realised by programmes which are planned to meet your individual needs and capacities.

f Reversibility

Your level of fitness will retrogress when you stop exercising. After only two weeks of inactivity, significant reductions of capacity can be measured and almost all training improvements are lost within several months. Many top athletes are in poorer physical condition several years after they retire from active sport, if they have not followed some other exercise programme, than the 50 year old executive who has played squash on a regular basis.

Control of exercise intensity

Your teacher must keep the intensity of the workout within your capacity. Monitoring of the pulse rate is probably the most convenient way of doing this, for jogging and other aerobic activities.

You should also familiarise yourself with the warning signs which may be indications of over-exercising, for example, excessive heart rate, deep breathing, pale skin and flushness. If you show any of these signs you should exercise at a reduced level, until you develop the capacity to handle more intensive exercise.

While these signs indicate the need for modifying the intensity of your activity, they are not signs of imminent danger. There *are* signs which do indicate danger, and if they appear, it means that exercise should be stopped immediately. These are:

1 Laboured breathing (difficulty with breathing, not the deep breathing normally associated with exercise).
2 Loss of co-ordination.
3 Dizziness.
4 Tightness in the chest.
5 Heat stress can be very dangerous and can occur in the gymnasium as well as out in the sun. You may suffer from any or all of the above symptoms if heat stress is being felt.

If any of these signs occur, exercise should not be continued until medical advice is obtained.

A flexible approach to exercise to music classes

1 A class may last for an hour rather than 45 minutes, and may have some advanced students who are capable of working for $1\frac{1}{2}$ hours. Provided that the basic components are dealt with, and that the class starts with a warm-up and ends with a cool-down, it can easily be adapted to last longer.
2 The shortening or lengthening of the aerobic, muscular strength and endurance or stretching components, are also quite acceptable. There may be a need in a class which has predominance of dancers, for the stretching component to be much longer. Provided that the teacher outlines to the participants the consequences of this change, and that each component naturally follows the other, then a change like this is quite acceptable.
3 The order of the components may be changed as shown in the graphs opposite.
4 Because of the 'plateauing' effect, it is quite acceptable for a class

to remain at a particular level for two or more weeks before progressing.

5 As you adapt and progress more of your class can be used intensively until finally the whole of the time is being used to the maximum. When you are able to sustain aerobic training for 20 minutes, a satisfactory level of fitness will have been reached. Your programme has now changed from a fitness *producing* programme to a fitness *maintaining* programme and you should now aim to exercise at least three times per week.

Planning a beginners' programme

The graphs below show the basic structure of two beginners' classes and a progression over 10 weeks. For the purposes of this beginners' programme, we will consider four of the components of a class, i.e. warm-up, aerobic, muscular strength and endurance and cool-down. The fifth component, stretching, will be included in both the warm-up and cool-down. We would recommend that beginners exercise like this three times a week for 45 minutes each time.

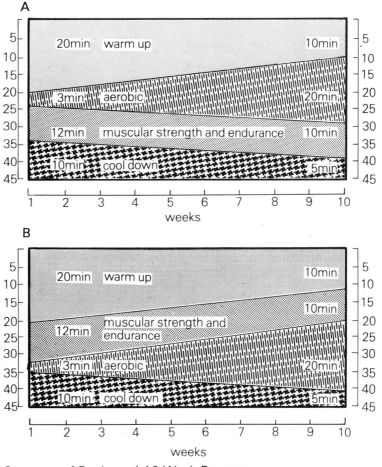

Structure of Beginners' 10 Week Programme

The graphs provide safe guidelines. The choice of either A or B will depend upon the teacher's preference and her assessment of the students capabilities.

It would be acceptable and appropriate to start with structure A for the first five or six weeks and then change to structure B for the rest of the ten week course.

During the early weeks of both plans a greater amount of time is devoted to the warm-up. In the case of some beginners, the simple warm-up exercises may prove to be enough for the cardio-respiratory systems. Consequently it would be more advisable for these beginners to follow on with a strength component rather than an aerobic component as in B.

In the first two or three weeks, time is spent learning exercises and routines and therefore natural breaks for demonstrations explanation give you time to recover. Naturally, as the ten week course progresses pupils will be capable of exercising more fully. Each component should be progressed using 3 principles of training: duration, frequency and intensity in order to gradually increase the exercise demand. The time allotted to each component will need to change in order for it to be a fully effective class by the tenth week, but it is important for your teacher to set you objectives at the beginning and for you to aim to achieve these by the end of the programme.

Controversial Exercises

Not every exercise can be performed by all individuals.

Different body types provide natural obstacles for some exercises and sporting activities. This is often overlooked not only by performers but also by teachers and coaches as well.

In Russia searches are made for the perfect body type for each sporting activity and great care is taken to provide an individual training programme for each chosen athlete.

Almost any exercise can be harmful if done incorrectly. Exercise to music is a programme for a wide cross-section of the public, not only top athletes. Consideration must be given to the level of fitness and basic working order of the untrained body. When careful thought is given to individual characteristics, it is not surprising that the teacher has a responsibility constantly to remind the participants to be careful if they have a bad back, weak joints, poor posture, weak muscles etc. and that everybody should avoid any exercise which hurts.

However, there are particular exercises that have been performed for years that are now thought to be harmful and can produce injury. The following exercises most frequently cause concern and we recommend that you do not do the exercises illustrated in this chapter:

Toe Touches

This is usually performed as a ballistic 'hamstring stretch'. However, this exercise forces the knees to over-extend and places a tremendous amount of pressure on the lumber vertebrae SP. (lower back). This is believed by many authorities to have an adverse effect on the lower back. However, if performed as a static stretch with knees slightly bent, to take the pressure off the lower back, it can be acceptable as an exercise but you must be aware of potential hazards.

Alternative Exercise
An alternative 'hamstring' (or back of the legs) stretch is performed by lying on the back grasping the extended leg at the knee and pulling it gently towards the chest. The other leg should be bent with the foot flat on the floor (see page 73.).

Toe touches
Causes strain on the lower back.

Avoid this exercise.

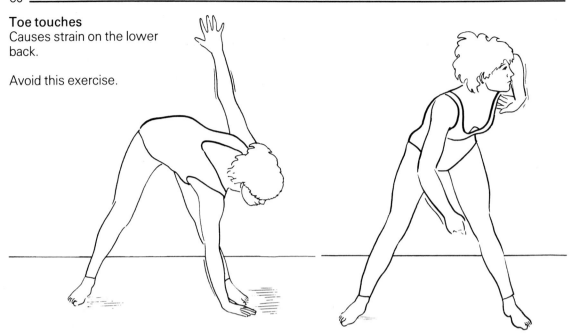

Straight Leg Sit-ups, Double Leg Raises

The straight leg sit-up is often done to 'strengthen the abdominals' but it is not as effective as it might be because of the action of the muscles which flex the hip joint. It is these muscles, i.e. the hip flexors, which are mainly used when a person 'sits up' with legs extended.

Furthermore there is a 'pull' on the spinal column when you sit up from this position which can cause a hyper-extension of the back placing undue stress on the lower spine.

Straight leg sit-ups
Causes strain on the lower back.

Avoid this exercise.

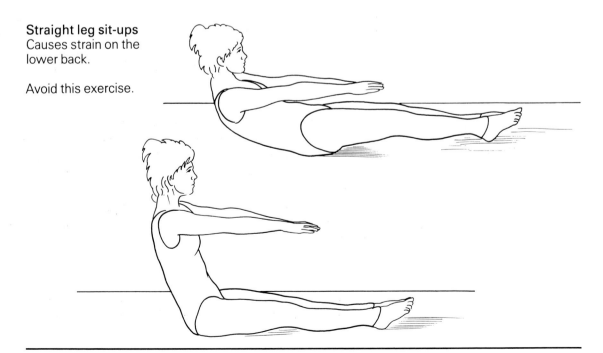

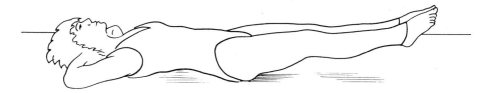

Double leg raises
Causes strain due to the arch in the lower back.

Avoid this exercise.

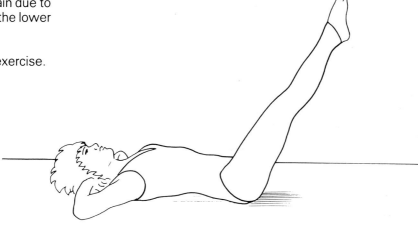

Alternative Exercise
Do your sit-ups with bent knees, i.e. lie on your back with knees bent and feet flat on the floor. Place your palms on the thighs and lift the shoulders slowly from the floor, sliding the palms up the thigh until they curl around the knees. Pause, then lower the shoulders only to the ground.

When doing leg raises, only one leg should be lifted at a time, while the other leg is bent with the sole of the foot flat on the floor. When doing either of these alternative exercises, you should pull in your abdominal muscles and force the small of the back into the floor.

Deep Knee Bends (full squats)

This is usually performed as a 'quads' or thigh strengthening exercise. However, forceful deep squatting stretches the ligaments of the knee. If the stretching is excessive the natural protection of the knee is all but eliminated. In some instances the cartilage of the knee can be pinched by deep squatting. Deep knee bends and 'duck walk' activities have been almost universally condemned by exercise physiologists. With these movements, ligaments can be stretched and thus the knee loses its stability and is predisposed to injury.

Alternative Exercise
The safest procedure would seem to be to squat only to the point where the thighs are parallel to the floor, and to eliminate all 'bouncing' squat movements, such as 'bunny hops'.

Deep knee bends
Puts strain on the knees.

Avoid this exercise.

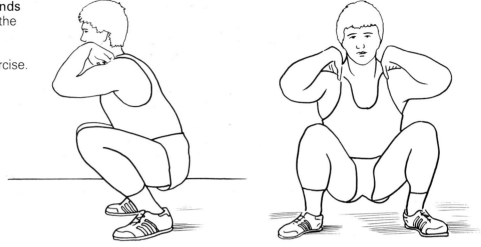

Hands Behind Head Sit-ups

Many people, when doing sit-ups, place their hands behind and around the neck or head and try to pull up the upper body by yanking on the hands. This can be potentially dangerous because of the undue pressure that is placed upon a delicate and vulnerable part of the upper spinal column.

Puts strain on the neck.

Avoid placing hands behind head.

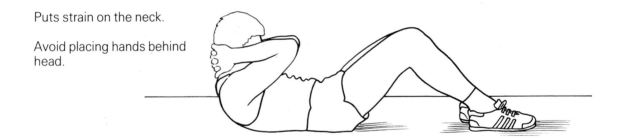

Alternative Exercise
Place the hands at the side of the face and over the ears or on the shoulders. It has also been suggested that for Senior Citizens, because of the weight of the head, that one hand be placed behind the head to support it and the other hand on the thigh.

ADDITIONAL CONSIDERATIONS WHEN CHOOSING EXERCISES
Head and Neck

Movements in this area *must* be slow and gentle and the range of movement never forced. Head and neck exercises should be undertaken only after loosening the shoulder girdle and the head should not be allowed to go too far back. Complete head circling, therefore, is not an exercise we would recommend you to do.

Alternative Exercise
Turn the head to the right, back to the centre and then to the left. Repeat as necessary.

Chin to chest, looking straight ahead, lift the chin up without forcing the head back.

Turn the head to the right, roll down the chin until the head is turned to the left. Repeat as necessary.

Back

Great care should be taken never to force extension, lateral flexion, forward flexion or rotation of the spine. Bouncing, pulling over, reaching or jerking can place an abnormal strain on the lower spine or create weaknesses of the joints or surrounding muscles.

When bending forwards with a flat back it is advisable to bend the knees and pull the stomach in to take the strain off the lower back. It has been found that a high number of back problems often occur from bending forward with a flat back and then twisting to the right or left.

Avoid these exercises

Flat back
Twisting with a flat back strains the lower back.

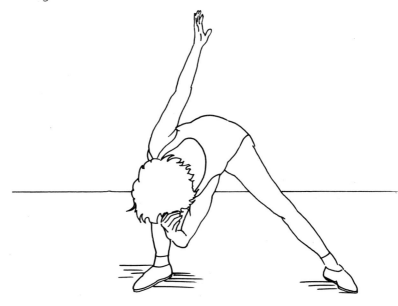

Extended arms adds to the danger.

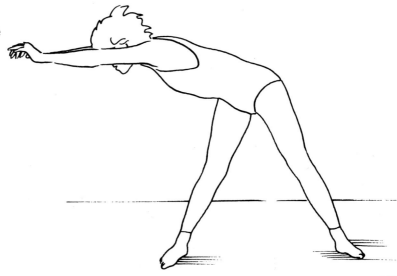

Tail or Coccyx

Some people have longer 'tails' than others, so care should be taken not to bounce or bang this area hard on the floor. When sitting on the end of the spine plenty of cushioning is needed, for example, from a mat. Moving from lying on the back to sitting can be uncomfortable for students with a long coccyx.

Lunge
Remember to keep both feet flat on the floor at all times.

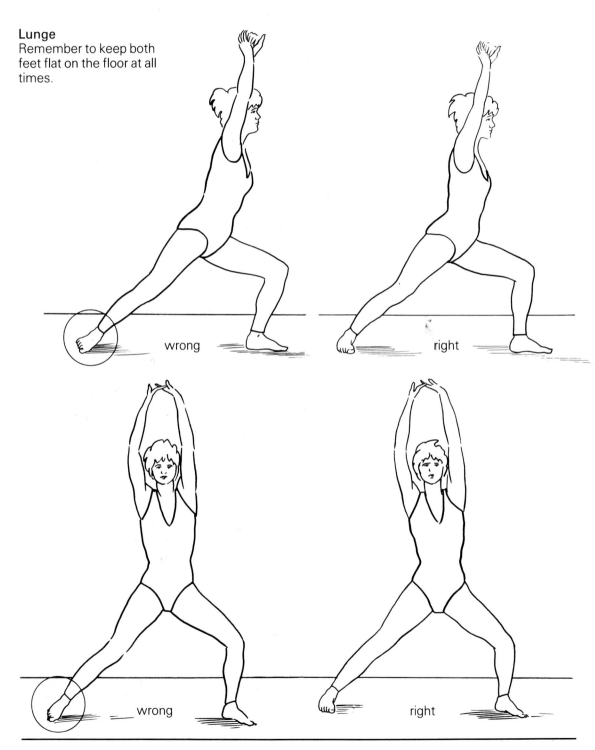

wrong

right

wrong

right

Jogging on the Spot

Jogging on the spot encourages jogging on the toes, which can cause shin splints and stress fractures in the leg and foot.

Alternative Exercises
You can reduce the amount of jogging on the spot, and increase the movement around the exercise area, emphasising the heel-toe action.

You can make sure that your heel is in greater contact with the floor thereby reducing the amount of force on the toes. If you 'give' at the knees this will also absorb the shock caused by your body weight coming down on the toes.

Avoid:

1 Performing exercises that are too fast and without muscle control.
2 Too many repetitions of any one exercise, thereby overworking one group of muscles or one joint.
3 Jerky or bouncing exercises.
4 Forcing any movement.
5 Over exertion if you are overweight, or underweight, very unfit, or have high blood pressure and heart trouble.
6 Weight-bearing exercises if you have stiff or bad joints, poor posture, weak muscles or a protruding belly.
7 Too strenuous exercise after operations, poor health, breaks or strains, post/ante-natal depression, illness, or old age.
8 Any exercise with a bent knee position where the knee is not above the foot.
9 The two lunge positions shown opposite unless the foot of the straight leg is flat to the floor. This avoids undue stress on the knee of the straight leg.
10 Placing the weight over the little toe when doing heel raises. If you keep the weight over the big toe it will prevent undue strain on the outside of the ankle (see below).

Heel raises
Keep weight over the big toe.

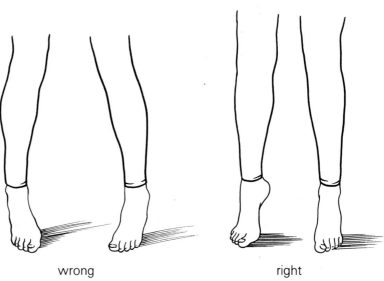

wrong   right

You Should Remember:	1 Not to wear slippery footwear.
	2 Not to wear tight clothing.
	3 Not to exercise when feeling unwell.
	4 Not to exercise on a full stomach or to chew gum while exercising.

A Good Exercise to Music Teacher will Always:

1 Refuse to accept as members of the class those 30% overweight or those under seven stone, without their doctor's written permission.
2 Constantly remind those who have or may have had a bad back to be careful; the golden rule is to avoid any exercise which hurts.
3 Check your starting position of an exercise and make sure your body is comfortable.
4 Enlist the help of any professional members of your group i.e. physiotherapist.
5 Remember that as a constant exerciser, they are much fitter than most of their class.

Partner Exercises

These should never be forced or hurried. Partners should be sympathetic to each others physical limitations. Everyone should work within their own range of movement.

WHEN YOU EXERCISE:

There should be no pain involved.

You should listen and feel the messages from your body and take heed.

You should never become exhausted.

10 Safety Concerns

An awareness of the potential hazards will enable you to enjoy your class to the full, secure in the knowledge that you are prepared for most eventualities and can avoid many of the problems before they occur.

Some of the safety concerns below may have been mentioned in other chapters. We believe that they all bear repeating time after time and so do not apologize to you for having to read some of them a second time.

You should be aware of:

1 Any medical problems which might cause you pain whilst exercising.
2 Signs of over-exertion and over-exercise such as:
   a Undue fatigue during exercise.
   b Inability to sleep at night.
   c Inability to recover from a workout throughout the day.
   d Persistent muscle aches and pains.
   e Failure of your pulse to return to 20 beats per minute over the resting heart rate after cool-down.
3 Signs indicating that you should stop exercising:
   a Laboured breathing or a difficulty in breathing, not the expected deep breathing normally associated with exercise.
   b Loss of co-ordination.
   c Dizziness.
   d Tightness in the chest or pain related to teeth, arm, jaw, ear or upper back.
   e Nausea or vomiting.
   f Irregular heart rate following exercise.
   g Muscular-skeletal problems aggravated by exercise.
   h Unusual weight loss.
4 Emergency procedures at the exercise site, where the telephones are located and the address of the nearest hospital's Out-Patients Department.
5 How to adjust your workout to accommodate daily and seasonal differences in temperature and humidity.
6 The correct clothing to wear; it should not be of a heat-retaining nature, i.e. sweat suits, sauna suits.
7 The correct footwear to wear; it should be supportive and

cushioning, while still allowing movement of the foot, forwards, backwards and sideways.

8 Pulse-taking methods and how to adjust your programme accordingly.

9 The state of your exercise floor; that it is dry and free from obstructions.

10 Your insurance cover in the event of an injury during exercise and that it is adequate.

NB: YOU SHOULD BEWARE OF TEACHERS WHO MAKE OR SUGGEST A MEDICAL DIAGNOSIS OR PRESCRIPTION UNLESS OF COURSE THEY ARE MEDICALLY QUALIFIED.

GENERAL PROCEDURES IN THE EVENT OF INJURY OR ACCIDENT

It is advisable for you to check that your teacher has attended a recognised course in First Aid. If this is the case you will probably be in good hands if you should have an accident.

Nevertheless, we list below certain steps that should be taken in the event of an injury or accident. Reading this section does not mean that you are now an authority in any sense of the word. The list is merely a guide to follow in an emergency, if there is not a competently trained person available and after you have sent someone to telephone for an ambulance.

1 Do not move the person.
2 Keep the person lying down whenever possible.
3 If the injured party is conscious, try to find out if she can feel pain.
4 If the injured party is unconscious, check breathing, pulse and for bleeding.
5 Look for injuries and do what first aid you can.
6 Give as much reassurance as you can. Give no statements concerning injuries to the injured party.

Wounds

1 Wash with water.
2 Apply a dressing if applicable.
3 Lightly bandage with gauze.
4 In the case of a puncture with a nail or a cut with a piece of metal, be sure to tell the person to get a Tetanus injection if she has not had one within the last year.
5 Do not remove foreign bodies from wounds.

Bleeding

1 Apply direct pressure with the hand. Use gauze if it is readily available as this will decrease the chances of infection.
2 Elevate the portion of the body that is bleeding.

Nose Bleed

1 This could be the result of an injury or an underlying disease such as hypertension.
2 Have the person tip their head forwards and pinch their nostrils between the fingers with gauze.
3 Do not alow the injured person to exercise further.
4 Do not allow blowing of the nose for 4 hours.

Shock	1 The symptoms are: dull eyes, dilated pupils, shallow and irregular breathing, weak or no pulse, pale clammy skin, nausea, sweat around the lips, forehead and armpits.
Diabetes	1 The common symptoms are: sweet, fruity breath, dry warm skin and rapid weak pulse. The person may become suddenly faint and confused and eventually lapse into coma. This can be caused by low blood sugar or too much Insulin. The injured party should be given glucose tablets, a glucose drink, or something which contains sugar as soon as possible.
Eye Injuries	1 Do not remove anything from the eyes. 2 For injuries, cover both eyes, and send the person to the hospital immediately. 3 For a black eye, apply ice as soon as possible.
Heart Attack	1 The symptoms are: shortness of breath, chest pain, blue colour of lips and finger nails, pain in shoulder and left arm, tightness in chest. 2 Make the person as comfortable as possible. If necessary, administer cardiopulmonary resuscitation and ensure an ambulance is called immediately.
Stroke	1 There are various symptoms, depending upon the severity of the attack, e.g. unconsciousness, heavy breathing, paralysis of upper or lower arm, pupils unequal in size. 2 Ensure an ambulance is called immediately.
Fainting	1 This is a reaction of the nervous system that results in a reduction in temperature or blood supply to the brain. 2 Put the head of the injured party between her knees to prevent passing out.
Unconscious	1 If unconscious, lie the injured party in the recovery position, preferably with legs raised. If consciousness does not return ensure an ambulance is called. 2 Loosen tight clothing.
Epilepsy	1 Loosen clothes and lie the person down in an open space so that she cannot hurt herself in her convulsions. 2 Do not restrain. 3 Do not put your fingers or anything else in the person's mouth. 4 Person is unusually sleepy after seizure. 5 Keep person quiet or another attack may occur.

POTENTIAL INJURIES: PREVENTION AND BASIC TREATMENT

All sport and physical activities involve some sort of physical stress, sometimes applied to the whole body and at other times to only parts of it. However, when sudden or excessive stress is applied to a particular part of the body, the force generated may exceed tolerable loads and injury may occur.

You should be aware of the dividing line between what is safe, and what is dangerous.

You cannot be expected to become an expert on sports injuries just because you take part in exercise to music classes. It is possible, however, for you to avoid many injuries by acquiring knowledge of factors affecting prevention and cause of injury, and to be aware of some basic remedial treatment.

A great deal of information in this chapter can be deduced from applying the knowledge from all of the previous chapters in this book. In some ways, it can be seen as a summation, or at least an adaption of much of the information.

PREVENTION OF INJURY

1 FITNESS

You must introduce yourself progressively and gradually to exercise. If you are overweight, have poor muscle tone, a lack of flexibility and your body is not accustomed to exercise, you are extremely vulnerable to injury.

2 WARM-UP AND COOL-DOWN

When you exercise you should warm up your body thoroughly before subjecting it to any work load. Blood should be circulating well into the muscles to warm them and joints should be fully mobilised. Your body should feel warm, loose and supple. At the end of an exercise class there will be large amounts of blood in the muscles, which if you stop suddenly may 'pool', particularly in the legs, and you may faint; hence the importance of a graduated cool-down.

3

As an individual, your level of cardiorespiratory fitness, amount of strength and endurance, and degree of flexibility will be unique. You should not be encouraged by others, or motivate yourself beyond your particular level of fitness. Your use of heart-rate monitoring can help to guide you to the level at which you should work.

4 INCORRECT EXERCISES

You should avoid controversial exercises or those which cause pain when you try to do them. At the same time, you should ensure that you perform even simple exercises correctly at all times.

FACTORS INFLUENCING INJURIES

1 FITNESS LEVEL

Violent exercise for the non-exerciser can be fatal. Even mild exercise for the unprepared body can cause painful injury. You should remember that fitness is specific. Because you are a very strong weight lifter does not mean that you could sustain a twenty minute aerobic session in an exercise to music class. Because you attend an exercise to music class three times a week, do not assume that you could run a half marathon.

2 PHYSIQUE AND BODY COMPOSITION

Do not expect miracles from your exercise class. Accept your somatotype and seek to improve it; do not expect to change it. Remember that if you are overweight you are more vulnerable to injury because of the extra force that your excess weight places on the joints, muscles and the circulatory system.

3 BAD POSTURE

Bad posture is aesthetically displeasing, potentially injurious and mechanically inefficient. Posture refers to the relative alignment of the body parts, in particular the head, spine, pelvic tilt and the feet. Body segments are balanced one upon the other and supported by the muscles. Hence, a slumped position decreases the volume within the body so that breathing requires greater effort, and the organs concerned with digestion are constricted and less efficient. Secondly, the joints experience unnecessary stress and strain and this may cause deterioration in old age, such as bow legs and 'rolled in' ankles. Postural faults can develop at birth or throughout life. The natural curve of the back when viewed from the side may become accentuated.

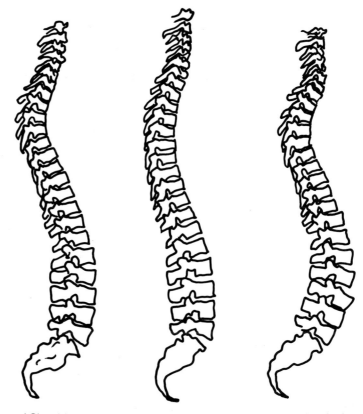

Round Shoulders   Correct   Lumbar Lordosis

a An over emphasis of the curve in the lumbar region may lead to a fault called *lordosis*, where the pelvis tilts the wrong way and the contents of the abdomen tip forward. The upper back tends to arch to balance the forward tilt, thus putting too great a stress on the lumbar vertebra.

b An increased curve in the thoracic region leads to round shoulders and an unattractive hunched-back appearance.

c A sideways curve in the back can also occur for those who overtrain one side of the body, for example, the hotel porter who always carries heavy luggage in the same hand or throwers in athletics.

Good posture is characterized by poise and control in movement. It is obvious whether you are standing, sitting, lying or moving and is maintained largely unconsciously by neuromuscular co-ordination. Nevertheless, posture can be improved by conscious effort:

a By improving the muscle tone and muscular strength and endurance.

b By improved flexibility, which will decrease the resistance in movement and therefore the tension created by stiff joints and muscles.

c By practice and a concentration on good posture.

4 TECHNIQUE

You should look for excellence in your technique while at the same time remembering that with an increase of fatigue there is usually a decrease in technique and, therefore a vulnerability to injury caused through poor technique.

5 ENVIRONMENT

Your exercise environment may put you at risk. Obstructions on a gym floor or protrusions from a gym wall may cause serious injury. Remember that a hot, humid environment, made worse by a large number of people exercising and producing heat in a room, will put the cardiovascular system under a certain amount of stress as it seeks to off-load your own body heat. Conversely, a cold environment will make you vulnerable to muscle strains and tears, and therefore you will need a longer warm-up.

6 AGE

As you get older, you deteriorate physiologically. Your cardiovascular system is less efficient and you have a lower maximum heart rate. Therefore, you are more prone to cardiorespiratory problems as well as ligament and tendon injuries, which will take longer to heal. Bones may become more brittle and arthritis more common.

Conversely, the young are still in the developmental stage and their bones, muscles and tendons may be extremely vulnerable. Care should be taken to ensure they are not placed under too much stress.

7 GENDER

You should remember that there are certain fundamental, anatomical and physiological differences between men and women. While not wishing to fall into the trap of over-emphasising these differences, we would be negligent if we did not mention them. In general terms, for example, men are stronger, faster and more powerful while women are more flexible.

COMMON TISSUE DAMAGE AND TREATMENT
Skin
1 ABRASION (GRAZE)

This occurs when layers of tissue, richly supplied with blood, are torn away and can be particularly painful as the nerve endings are exposed.

Treatment: Abrasions should be gently cleaned with mild antiseptic, and an oily or non-stick dressing should be applied.

2 CONTUSION (BRUISE)

This is caused when internal bleeding occurs after the tissue in the skin is torn.

Treatment: An ice-pack should be applied as soon as possible.

3 LACERATION (CUT)

Depending upon the severity of the cut, it should be closed either by dumbell plasters or stitches after efforts have been made to clean the wound and avoid infection.

4 BLISTERS

These are caused by friction when one layer of skin is detached from the underlying layer, the gap being filled by watery fluid from the injured cells, and can be painful when the outer layer is lifted and the nerve endings exposed.

Treatment: The fluid should be released by means of a needle which has been sterilised by being heated in a flame and then quenched immediately in spirit or water. Cover the wound with a zinc oxide plaster or dry dressing extending well beyond the blister.

Muscles

1 *Intrinsic* damage is caused when there is a tear or a strain of the muscle. This is probably caused by a co-ordination problem or over-stretching.
2 *Extrinsic* damage is caused by a direct blow on a muscle.
3 A *Haematoma*, or bleeding within the muscle, is caused when blood escapes into the surrounding tissues, causing a rise in the tension and pain when the muscle is contracted. Eventually the blood works its way to the surface of the skin producing a discolouration or bruise, although not always at the place one would expect.

Treatment: Rest, Ice, Compression and Elevation, which can be easily remembered by the initial letters ICE.
This treatment should be immediate.

ICE

Ice numbs the damaged area and works as an analgesic, causing the constriction of the blood vessels to that area, quickly reducing the bleeding into the damaged area. The early application of ice, not directly to the skin but in a polythene bag or towel, will prevent the excessive bleeding, most of which occurs in the first few minutes after injury.

COMPRESSION

Immediate bandaging, evenly and not too firmly applied, will also prevent further bleeding.

ELEVATION

Following injury, the *venous return*, or the process by which the blood is returned to the heart, is reduced. There is a tendency therefore, for the blood and tissue fluid to 'pool' in the damaged muscle and limb. Elevating the damaged limb will allow gravity to supplement the venous return.

Tendons

Even though tendons are very strong, they can be sprained or ruptured. If the achilles tendon ruptures it feels like you have been struck a blow and sounds like the crack of a whip. With peritendinitis, there is inflammation and swelling, caused by over-use of the tendon and its surrounding sheath. After exercise, a dull ache is felt, there is swelling at the site and pain in the area over the tendon when it is touched.

Treatment: ICE and rest.

Ultrasound can be used by a physiotherapist. Steroid injections or anti-inflammatory drugs can be administered by a doctor.

Joints

1 Swelling at a joint is usually caused by weeping from the synovial membrane.
2 Stiffness in the joint could mean that the muscles are 'in spasm', a protective mechanism of the body. You should not use any force to try to bend or straighten the joint.
3 Spraining of the joint can mean damage to the ligaments and capsule, caused by a movement beyond its normal range.
4 Dislocation. The extent of the damage may be revealed by comparing it with the same joints on the opposite limb.

Treatment: The joints should be rested either by a sling, strapping or plaster, all of which will normally be applied by a doctor.

With some joint injuries the attached muscle may be exercised to maintain tone and strength and help absorption of the tissue fluid.

Bones

Stress fractures in bones can be compared with fatigue fracture in metal. Over-exercising or incorrect footwear in exercise to music classes may cause fractures.

If the following symptoms are evident a doctor should be consulted.

1 Variable but sharp and severe pain, swelling and bruising.
2 Slight deformity of the bone.
3 The bone is tender to the touch.
4 Pressure cannot be exerted by either pulling or pushing.
5 A grating noise can be heard during movement.

SOME COMMON INJURIES
Lower Leg

'Shin Splints' or a pain in the front of the leg, with the bone tender to the touch, is quite common in exercise to music classes. It could be caused by a number of different conditions:

1 A stress fracture of the fibula.
2 Inflammation of the periosteum, caused by a pull on the periosteum along the edge of the tibia.
3 The anterior libeal muscle, lying in a compartment between the tibia and the fibula, can become tight and suffer from a reduced blood supply.

Treatment: Ice, ultrasound, heel raises when the pain is reduced, flexibility work on the calves and strengthening exercises on the front of the lower leg.

Knee Joint

Damage to the knee joint is one of the most common joint injuries. It may be caused by:

1 A torn cartilage and, if so, you can hear a 'click' in the knee.
2 Torn or pulled cruciate ligaments which normally stabilise the knee by their 'cross-like' structure.
3 Pulled or torn medial and lateral ligaments.
4 A softening of the cartilage of the knee cap. The patella moves and twists over the bottom of the femur approximately 800 times when you run a mile. The cartilage behind the knee cap or patella can become roughened, inflamed, swollen and quite painful.

Treatment: Rest, ice, exercising the 'quads' and a visit to a physiotherapist.

Foot

1 There are many small bones that may be injured in the foot. For example, a stress fracture, or 'march fracture' of the metatarsals.
2 If there is inflammation of the protective plantar fascia on the underside of the foot, you will have a dull ache in the heel.

Treatment: Rest, padding to support the foot, and muscle strengthening exercises.

Foot and Ankle

1 The most common injury in the whole of sport is a sprain of the lateral ligament which can become swollen, very painful and often give indication of a fracture.
2 If the ligaments which hold the ankle joints together are torn, surgery is often the only treatment.
3 Occasionally, the edges of the bones of the ankle can be detached. Surgery is the only cure.

Treatment: ICE followed by a visit to the physiotherapist.

Spinal Injuries

Isolating the exact injury to the spine can be problematic as many are possible, for example:

1 Damage to the ligaments of the spine.
2 Damage to the muscles supporting the spine.
3 Inflammation of the bones or cartilage.
4 Abnormalities of the blood supply to the spine.
5 Infections of the spine.
6 Damage to the discs or nerves of the spine, which can often cause pain either in the leg or arm.

If you are unfortunate and sustain an injury that enables you to function in general terms, but prevents you from following your exercise programme, you should consult your doctor as soon as possible. Quite often your doctor will not have the time to give you a great deal of attention, and you should ask her to refer you to a chartered physiotherapist, who specialises in this kind of injury and rehabilitation from it.

Nutrition

Nutrition is an area beset by inaccurate information, faddism, obsession, trendiness, massive commercial interests, and subject to the whole force of multi-media advertising. The truth is hard to find amid the welter of enlightened self-interest and deception.

In general terms the body requires a variety of thirty or forty different types of food in order to supply the body tissues with certain essential nutrients.

PROTEIN

Protein provides energy for growth and the repair of tissues, and is found in eggs, cheese, milk, fish, meat, lentils, peas, beans and nuts.

CARBOHYDRATE

Carbohydrate breaks down into sugar and provides energy quite quickly, which if not needed immediately is stored as fat. It is found in bread, sweets, sugar, potatoes, pasta and rice.

FAT

Fat, from either vegetable or animal sources, provides energy or is stored as fat, and serves as insulation for the body. It is found in margarine, butter, cream, fat from meat, milk, cheese and nuts.

WATER

Water provides the fluid that is vital to the body. We can survive without food for long periods, but cannot survive for long without water.

VITAMINS AND MINERAL SALTS

Vitamins and mineral salts are essential for good health. A balanced diet will provide in normal circumstances, all that the body needs without the necessity for additives. There should be no need for a special diet, which should only be followed after medical advice.

The need for a special 'balanced diet' has, in the past, usually referred to nutritional problems caused by a lack of vital nutrients, particularly in children, pregnant women, the elderly, or those on very low incomes. At the present time in the western world there are very few who, through lack of resources, suffer from vitamin deficiency. Today's nutritional problems, however, are caused by an unbalanced diet due to eating too much of certain types of food and insufficient of others:

1 Too much saturated fat increases your calorie intake and can lead to deposits of fatty substances on the inner lining of the arteries, which can cause heart disease.

2 Too much sugar increases your calorie intake and can cause tooth decay, gallstones and diabetes.

3 Too much salt tends to raise the blood pressure and increase the incidence of heart disease and strokes.

4 Too many calories increase your weight and can increase the risk of high blood pressure, diabetes and heart disease.

5 Eating too little fibre can slow down the digestive processes and cause bowel disorders.

Good nutrition should essentially be common sense. The nutrients that you need are available quite naturally in many types of food and at a reasonable cost. There is very little gain in paying for expensive health foods and additives. It is possible to eat things you like and still lose weight; you are able to improve your fitness without eating half a dozen assorted vitamin products; you can be healthy without restricting your food intake to only four or five types of food.

Nutrition and Energy/Fuel

A basic energy requirement to enable you to exist is about 1200 calories a day. An average intake should be around 2,500 calories per day, although this figure is lower for women than for men of the same body weight. This energy intake is usually made up of:

1 45% from carbohydrates, of which typically 60% is from sugars and 40% from starch.

2 45% from fats, of which typically 75% comes from animal sources, saturated fats, and 25% from vegetable sources, unsaturated fats.

3 The remaining 10% comes largely from protein and alcohol, with 50% protein coming from animal sources and 50% from vegetable sources.

Any energy not used is stored as fat. If you remember that a half marathon run uses only 1,300 calories you might be inclined to abandon, in despair, your exercise programme. However, *regular* exercise speeds up your metabolic rate, i.e. the rate at which you naturally burn up calories. Therefore regular exercise combined with sensible eating will enable you to lose weight, stay healthy and improve your shape.

Recently a group of reputable academic experts produced the NACNE Report (The National Advisory Council for Nutritional Education). The recommendations constitute sound advice and should be followed.

1 Restrict your energy intake to prevent energy being stored as fat; in this way you will maintain your body weight and avoid obesity, which can be a health hazard.

2 Start to exercise or increase your exercise programme in order to use up your energy intake.
3 Reduce the percentage of fat contribution to energy from 45% to 30%.
4 Reverse the animal/vegetable proportions of your fat contribution to 25%/75%.
5 Increase your carbohydrate contribution to energy from 45% to 60% if possible.
6 Reduce the sugar proportion of your carbohydrate contribution.
7 Reduce the proportion from animal sources of your protein contribution.
8 Reduce the amount of added salt.
9 Increase the amount of fibre in your diet by 50%.

Even though we have recommended the NACNE Report to you, unfortunately even its recommendations have been bedeviled by controversy. Criticisms have been made which though unsound in nutritional terms, may be sound in economic and social terms. If everyone followed NACNE advice, the consumption of meat, milk, butter, cheese, etc. would be severely reduced, nutritionally a good thing. Those concerned with the production of these products in the farming industry would argue that hardship would be caused if this industry was adversely affected. Nevertheless, we would recommend the NACNE Report to you.

Exercise and Energy/Fuel

When one looks at fuels in our diet, and the fuels available and used in exercise, one is not looking at a simple equation.

1 Energy left over is stored as fat – a potential source of fuel.
2 Fuel is stored in the muscle as glycogen, which consists of carbohydrate units stacked together in long chains – exercise depletes this glycogen store.

When you exercise, you do not use only one fuel store. In running, for example, the fuel used is from both carbohydrate and fat stores, as indicated in the diagram below.

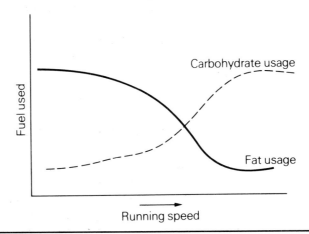

Carbohydrate usage

Fat usage

Fuel used

Running speed

When you walk you use fat stores as fuel. As your rate of exercise speeds up, the only way fuel can be produced fast enough is by using more and more from carbohydrate stores, which has a fast rate of conversion.

When you exercise regularly, the balance is changed, and fat stores will be used, sparing your *glycogen* stores. To some extent this is quite a significant fact because glycogen stores are limited and are also very small when one compares them to the enormous protein and fat stores, e.g.

Energy stores related to a usual diet

	Calories
Muscle glycogen	480
Liver glycogen	280
Protein	24,000
Fat	141,000

The store of calories in muscle and liver glycogen would be inadequate fuel to run a half marathon.

It is important, therefore, when you follow an exercise programme that you replace your glycogen levels by taking in adequate carbohydrates, preferably in the form of starch, and also have a rest day to allow the glycogen to return to its normal level. If you regularly exercise to music, therefore, you should increase the carbohydrate percentage of your daily intake and make sure you have a rest day to allow your body to replenish its glycogen stores. A high protein diet is not appropriate if you exercise regularly because of its slow rate of conversion to fuel used in exercise, and because its primary function is to promote energy for growth and the repair of tissue.

Exercise and Fluids

It is essential to maintain your body fluids when you exercise. As you exercise, your body heats up. If your fluid levels are low you will cease to lose body heat by sweating, your blood volume will go down and eventually you will collapse.

During prolonged exercise take in fluid.

After exercise your priority is first fluid, second carbohydrate.

Exercise and Sugar

Do not take sugar, or sugar additives, before or during exercise, as it can be very dangerous. Blood sugar levels are lowered because the following happens:

1 Fluid is drawn from the body into the gut, and dehydration occurs.
2 The body's insulin release mechanism switches off the body's fat metabolism, and causes glycogen to be used up more quickly.
3 The muscles are starved of glycogen, and take sugar from the rest of the body.
4 Muscles will fatigue, the body may dehydrate and stomach cramps set in – collapse may follow.

If you wish to exercise regularly and would like to lose weight, we would recommend the following approach:

1 Aim to lose only 1 kilogram per week.
2 Increase your carbohydrate intake and increase the percentage of starch.
3 Eat more fruit, vegetables and wholegrain cereals.
4 Do not add salt to your meals.
5 Have a high carbohydrate breakfast: e.g. muesli, toast, honey, fruit juice and tea.
6 Reduce your sugar consumption in general.
7 Reduce your fat intake by cutting out all visible fat and switching from dairy produce to low fat products.

12 Conclusion

We have set out to produce guidelines which will help you to gain the maximum benefit from your exercise to music classes. We have also tried to put exercise to music in its context as one of many types of exercise in which you can involve yourself. We have indicated the legitimate expectations you may have of your teacher and you should now be able to evaluate your teacher's competence.

You should also now be aware of why you should exercise and have some knowledge of what is happening to your body during exercise and you should be able to evaluate your own progress. Certain myths should now have been exploded, for example:

1 Women who perform strength exercises will grow large muscles.
2 Eating less is the best or only way to lose weight and improve your shape.
3 You are fit if you are healthy.
4 You are healthy if you are fit.
5 All teachers, because they are teachers, know best.
6 You have to really suffer in order to become fit.

On yet a more positive note, you should have enough knowledge to identify your own specific objectives which should be similar to the following:

1 To develop optimum cardio/vascular fitness, in order to delay the degenerative changes typically associated with physical inactivity.
2 To develop muscular strength and endurance and flexibility in order to meet adequately the demands placed on your body through work and recreation.
3 To develop flexibility of the joints, in order to ensure normal postural alignment and aid prevention of injury due to sudden strains.
4 To seek opportunities for relaxation and the release of physical and mental tension.
5 To develop an understanding of the contribution of physical activity to general good health, and a knowledge of the significance of different activities in fulfilling this role.

6 To seek further information in order to develop your knowledge and awareness of good exercise/health behaviour and ultimately to improve your lifestyle.

7 To enjoy yourself while you exercise.

You should view the information you have gained from this book only as the start in your task of acquiring knowledge about exercise and exercise programmes. It is up to you to develop your own ideas and to build upon the foundations which this book has given you. You should review regularly your own ideas about fitness, exercise and nutrition. This review should include new methods and ideas and reinforce the concept that fitness is not a fad but a way of life.

Recommended Reading

1 Anderson, Bob, *Stretching* (Pelham Books, second edition 1985).
2 Gillie, Oliver, Celia Haddon and Derrik Mercer (eds), *The Sunday Times New Book of Body Maintenance* (Mermaid Books, Michael Joseph Ltd 1982).
3 Hazeldine, Rex, *Fitness for Sport* (The Crowood Press 1985).
4 Kennedy, Pat, *The Moving Body* (Faber & Faber 1979).
5 Maryon-Davis, Alan and Jane Thomas, *Diet 2000 How To Eat for a Healthier Future* (Pan Books Ltd 1984).
6 *First Aid Manual*, The authorised manual of St John's Ambulance, St Andrew's Ambulance Association and The British Red Cross Society (Dorling Kindersley London 1982).
7 Williams, Melvin H. *Nutritional Aspects of Human Physical and Athletic Performance* (Thomas Publications 1976).
8 Read, Dr Malcolm and Paul Wade, *Sports Injuries* (Breslich & Foss 1984).
9 Rowett H G C, *Basic Anatomy and Physiology* (John Murray Publishers Ltd 1983).
10 Bassey E J and P H Fentem, *Exercise The Facts* (Oxford University Press 1981)

Index

Page numbers in *italic* refer to the illustrations